THE
24/7
BABY
DOCTOR

A Harvard Pediatrician Answers All Your Questions from Birth to One Year

VICTORIA ROGERS McEVOY, MD,
with Florence Isaacs

LYONS PRESS
Guilford, Connecticut
An imprint of Globe Pequot Press

*For Earl, the man who has always had
my back, in parenting and in life*

To buy books in quantity for corporate use
or incentives, call **(800) 962-0973**
or e-mail **premiums@GlobePequot.com**.

Lyons Press is an imprint of Globe Pequot Press

Text design: Sheryl P. Kober
Project Editor: Ellen Urban
Layout: Mary Ballachino

Library of Congress Cataloging-in-Publication Data
McEvoy, Victoria Rogers.
  The 24/7 baby doctor : a Harvard pediatrician answers all your questions from birth to one year / Victoria Rogers McEvoy ; with Florence Isaacs.
     p. cm.
  Includes bibliographical references.
  ISBN 978-0-7627-5335-2
 1. Infants—Care—Miscellanea. 2. Pediatrics—Miscellanea. I. Isaacs, Florence. II. Title.
  RJ61.M486 2010
  618.92′02—dc22

                                    2009046727

Printed in the United States of America
10 9 8 7 6 5 4 3 2 1

6/10 f

Contents

Introduction

When will my baby sleep through the night? What should I do if the baby has a cold? Is my baby eating enough? Should my baby be walking by now? How tall will my baby be? Does my baby have colic? What if the baby chokes? Can I hurt the baby's soft spot? Why do babies spit up? In more than thirty years as a practicing pediatrician, these are the kinds of questions new parents have asked me over and over again as they begin the journey through their baby's first year of life. It's likely you have many of the same questions—plus a list of new ones because raising a child today is more complex than ever before. New scientific knowledge, amazing technology, and societal changes have created issues that never existed in the past. Twenty years ago, parents didn't ask, "Should I buy organic?"

Day after day of well-baby visits and worried phone calls have given me a window into parents' very natural concerns. As a parent, you're probably awed by this tiny addition to the household, yet anxious about being on your own and coping with the intricacies of infant care and new responsibilities. It's daunting to be charged with keeping a helpless baby healthy and safe. Along with the incredible love and wonder of a new child comes the overwhelming need to protect.

You may be competent and successful at work, yet few if any of the skills you've mastered prepare you for your newest job—parenting a baby who is totally dependent on you. At the same time, it's hard to pick up a newspaper or watch the news today without being assaulted by reports of the latest toxins, infections, and other threats lurking in the shadows. My goal is to help guide you through the confusion and myriad worries by answering the most frequent questions new parents ask me. These questions cover sleep, breastfeeding, nutrition, crying, development, illness, and other issues that inevitably arise during baby's first year. In my experience, although parents are individuals with varying personalities and backgrounds, they share basic concerns. You probably worry about doing something wrong that could harm the baby—just like everyone else. "What if I drop him?" seems to be a universal fear. So is worry about whether and when to call the doctor, and how to know if the baby is sick. Many parents obsess about the baby's growth and whether their child is on track with milestones.

Because I have been on the front line of day-to-day parental interactions, I know the information necessary to calm you down when anxiety takes hold. My focus is on evidence-based facts and recommendations. Some fears can be addressed by data and research, such as, "Is it dangerous if the umbilical stump is bleeding?" Others cannot. For example, there is no surefire way to determine whether formula (versus breast milk) leads to obesity later in life. I've included plenty of pediatric wisdom as well, from my decades as a clinician and my own experiences as a mother and grandmother.

Much in the world of child-rearing is based on family tradition, conventional wisdom, personal opinion, and, sometimes, studies that are not always well-conceived—where variables may be uncontrolled and results dubious. The answers ahead will help you sift through the avalanche of information available today and separate current scientific knowledge from misleading hyperbole. The Internet is a valuable tool, but it can also confuse you about even the most basic principles of child care. The point is not to disregard new ideas and differing points of view, but rather to become a critical recipient of information.

What has also become clear to me is that scientific "truths" are subject to change, as we constantly discover more about the mysteries of the human body, treatments and medications, and disease prevention. In my clinical life, I have seen such certainties as "Babies must go to sleep on their stomachs to prevent aspiration" replaced by "Babies must sleep on their backs to prevent SIDS," due to new knowledge. There are many such shifts, and that's what medical progress is all about.

BE YOURSELF

I also hope to educate and empower you to act within your own parenting style. You may be in your element rocking your infant to sleep—while your friend feels useless unless she is cross-country skiing or on a bird-watching expedition with her baby. You may feel, "I could never stay home all day," even as your sister-in-law declares, "All the action is at home. I want to be here." There is no one way or right way to be a parent. There are many wonderful ways to raise children and, despite your fears to the contrary, you probably have great instincts. Try to respect and use them, leavened by common sense.

I've guided so many parents through their baby's first year, and then beyond. And in turn, parents have taught me that they bring an incredible number of strengths to their role. You and your spouse have your own unique talents. If you don't accept and value them, you may continually feel that you are falling short or failing. Be prepared that you're going to make mistakes along the way. Everyone does, and I've made many of my own. Fortunately even newborns are hardy little people who are quite forgiving. Stories of your "no harm done" first year missteps may even wind up as fodder for dinner party jokes, although they might not have seemed so funny at the time.

You will also learn what you can control—such as baby-proofing your home to prevent accidents—and what you cannot. "Will my baby be smart?" is a very common question. There is no answer, although there are many ways you can help stimulate cognitive development, such as talking to your baby as much as possible from birth. One-on-one interaction is a priceless gift you can give your child. Many physical characteristics, such as height and body frame, depend on the gene pool. Babies are individuals, as well, with their own personalities that add to the brew. For all these reasons, parenting is a humbling pursuit. Try to accept that truth and do your best to hang on to your sense of humor.

HOW TO USE THIS BOOK

This book is a tool that gives you quick, authoritative answers to your most pressing questions and concerns. It is not an encyclopedia nor is it meant to be read cover-to-cover in one sitting. Instead, I hope you will turn to appropriate chapters as needed for help in dealing with on-the-spot dilemmas, and to anticipate situations that you will likely encounter and want to learn more about. Certain predictable issues will arise as soon as your baby comes home from the hospital; others will emerge in later months as your baby grows and develops. Your life will be so much easier when you learn how to handle these challenges.

The early chapters cover the basics of getting the baby to sleep through the night; breastfeeding; starting off right with nutrition; coping with crying; assessing bowel movements, voiding, and spit ups; and understanding growth and development. Chapter 7 answers questions about your baby's body, including puzzling changes you may notice, conditions babies outgrow, and conditions that are permanent but harmless. Most of the time what parents fear is an abnormality is actually just a variation of normal. Chapter

8 focuses on daily care issues, such as the best UV protection for your baby. Chapter 9 covers immunizations and addresses concerns about autism. In Chapters 10 and 11 you'll learn how to handle common illnesses and injuries such as getting the baby's finger caught in the door. Chapter 12 discusses allergy concerns in the first year. Later chapters answer questions about assessing health information, dealing with career issues and balancing parenting, nurturing your marital relationship post-baby, and taking care of your own health when you're always on call.

WORKING AS A TEAM

Your role as a parent during this first year is going to exhaust and stress you at times, as well as bring new meaning to your life and unimaginable joy. When you've been up all night with a crying baby or you're feeling insecure about your ability to parent, it should come as no surprise that tensions may arise between you and your spouse. To help prevent or deal with conflict, each chapter includes a sidebar on *Talking Together.* You and your partner bring a unique mix of personal history and emotion to your parenting roles. Family heritage, life philosophy, cultural background, energy level, and emotional baggage can vary tremendously from one person to the next. The two of you will work together more effectively and minimize hurdles when you share feelings and discuss values, expectations, and goals. In forming an effective family unit, each voice should be heard. Both of you must have input into major family decisions.

I know you're both busy. But you don't think twice about spending hours choosing and buying baby equipment. Taking time to talk together is just as important, and it offers an extra bonus: deeper understanding of each other that brings you closer together. Identifying and appreciating your strengths allows each of you to do what you do best.

A BUSY YEAR

No parent is immune to worry—not even me. As a mother of four and now as a grandmother, I have had my share—beginning on day one when my oldest child, my daughter, was born. I know your concerns because I've been in the same position myself. It isn't easy to come to terms with the realization that you are actually in charge of this tiny person's life and well-being.

Such anxieties are part of the human condition. But the questions and answers ahead will help you weed out needless fears, cope with real concerns, and start good parenting habits rather than face the much harder task of breaking bad ones later. The question-and-answer format will also help you work productively with the doctor. Your pediatrician is your partner and consultant in keeping your baby happy, healthy, and growing. Your fit with the doctor is important. You're going to rely on her regularly in your baby's first year; you want to choose someone you trust and with whom you feel comfortable. For details on how to select or switch doctors, see Chapter 8.

This first year is a journey of growth and exploration for your baby, and an amazing learning experience for you and your partner. Remember to laugh and enjoy it—and to be the kind of loving parent that fits your philosophy and strengths.

CHAPTER 1

Sleep—Getting to ZZZs

This chapter covers:

- The safest sleeping location
- Starting a sleep routine
- Wake-ups and sleeping through the night
- Sleep equipment
- Sudden Infant Death Syndrome (SIDS)

Babies' sleep is the topic I talk most about with new parents when they come to my office. Sleep issues trump every other subject except illness, and they are likely to occupy your thoughts much of the time—with good reason. Nothing has a greater impact on your family's quality of life during those first few months. Part of my role is to reassure you that this is a natural period of adjustment for the entire household. Both you and the baby are getting to know each other, and it will take time to find a natural rhythm. The same baby that adds so much joy to your life is also a demanding little person. Until the baby sleeps through the night, nobody will get much rest, and you and your spouse are going to feel exhausted and frustrated.

Following are the most frequent questions parents ask me about sleep. The answers cover a wide range of concerns and will help you set the stage for healthy sleep habits.

DEMYSTIFYING SLEEP

Where should the baby sleep?

Parents have always had options for infants' sleeping arrangements. The baby could sleep in his own room (if you have the space), or in his own bed in your room, or in your bed with you (known as "the family bed" or "bed sharing").

But in recent years, the safety of some sleeping arrangements has come into question.

The safest sleeping environment is room sharing, where your infant sleeps in a separate crib in your bedroom. Research indicates that room sharing reduces the risk of Sudden Infant Death Syndrome (SIDS), the sudden unexplained death of an apparently healthy baby. I advise room sharing for at least the first four or five months, when SIDS is most likely to occur. You can then transition the baby to a separate room (if you have one) or a separate space.

What's wrong with a family bed?

Having a "family bed" or "bed sharing" is routine in certain countries, where everyone piles in. Bed sharing is also popular with some parents in the United States, and many studies suggest this arrangement supports breastfeeding and infant-mother bonding. However, epidemiological studies show that bed sharing can be dangerous, and may result in suffocation, or other dangers. Major worries are that a parent who is a deep sleeper, is exhausted, or has been drinking alcohol or taking medication will be less aware and may roll over on the infant; or that smothering might occur due to soft bedding; or that the baby's head might get wedged between the headboard and mattress.

How can I settle my baby into a sleep routine?

A new baby invariably turns the entire household upside down in the first weeks. Initially, a good night's sleep can seem like a faded memory. You're still learning the basics of infant care, and it will take time for the family to settle into some kind of routine. It's important to maintain that routine, whatever shape it takes, even though your baby's sleep schedule will change down the road. Babies require less sleep as they grow and develop.

Because each infant is unique, individual sleep patterns

vary tremendously. Your child's schedule may be very different from that of another infant. You can usually expect a routine to evolve within approximately four weeks.

The best sleep approach for a newborn (an infant up to two weeks old) differs from what's appropriate a few months later. Of course you're going to love and nurture your newborn. You're going to hold him, cuddle him, and walk him around. But as soon as you sense he's getting drowsy, put him down in the crib on his back (the safest position) before his eyes close. At first he may fuss a little, which is normal. Just give him a chance to settle himself, and he'll fall asleep. Do not make the mistake of letting a newborn regularly fall asleep on your chest or in your arms. If you let that become a routine, you'll regret it. As soon as you transfer the sleeping baby to the crib, he'll wake up and start screaming. Yes, there may be times when he dozes off in your arms before you realize it. There's no need to be concerned. The point is to avoid making a habit of it.

Can't I rock the baby to sleep in a rocking chair?

This is a cozy and fun experience. If you keep doing it, however, your infant won't nod off any other way. Rocking becomes a trap you're stuck with. That doesn't mean you have to give up the pleasure of rocking. Just enjoy it occasionally and keep it brief or you'll quickly begin to resent it. It's sweet to rock at 6:00 p.m., but you're apt to feel differently at 11:00 p.m. six months later. As soon as you see that the baby seems sleepy as you rock, get her into the crib. Expect some fussing before she gets to sleep. It will eventually stop. A little fussing now is better than three hours of bloodcurdling screams at nine months.

What if the baby falls asleep while nursing?

Here's a common scenario: You feed the baby in your bed and she falls asleep on top of you, sated. You and your spouse are too tired to move her back to the crib. Before you know it, she can only fall asleep in one position—on you. Babies like this spot and usually want to sleep on their stomach. They've been curled up like this in utero, and haven't fully adapted to life outside the womb.

You can head off this habit by putting the baby down in her bed on her back while she's sleepy, but still awake. Make this a ritual. Do it consistently every time and you lay the foundation for sleeping through the night later. Baby will quickly learn that the back is the position in which she goes to sleep.

How do I know if the baby is sleeping enough?

Some infants stay awake all day (aside from short catnaps) and then sleep for long periods at night. Others who are still exhausted from the birth process can sleep virtually around the clock, getting up only to feed every two or three hours. There are also infants who seem to be awake night and day. Their parents worry that they aren't sleeping enough. I've found that (assuming there is no medical problem) infants who have an opportunity to sleep and don't, just don't need the sleep. This pattern is temporary and will eventually change.

What can we do if the baby sleeps all day and is up all night?

If your baby seems destined to work the night shift, restrict daytime sleep to a maximum of three hours at a stretch to avoid confusion about night and day and establish a normal routine. On the other hand, babies should sleep as much as they want at night (after regaining their birth weight)—unless there are medical reasons why your pediatrician wants you to wake the baby sooner.

Do we have to tiptoe around while the baby is sleeping? How quiet does the room have to be?

It's actually better to get an infant accustomed to noise right at the start to avoid the "princess and the pea" syndrome, where the mildest disturbance wakes the baby. Feel free to vacuum; play music; do whatever you would usually do in your day-to-day life. You want your baby to adjust to the normal environment in your home, just as he will have to learn to function in all types of environments out in the world. Children do adjust, even under surprising circumstances. One mom recalls her sons' bedroom overlooked a major city thoroughfare where a fire engine or an ambulance or police car siren might shriek at any hour of the day and night. Her sons usually slept through the racket.

How should we handle middle of the night wake-ups?

It's normal for babies up to five months or so to wake for short intervals in the middle of the night. Crying newborns need to be picked up and comforted. They must know they can count on being acknowledged and consoled. After a few weeks, however, you can let the baby fuss for a while. Instead of rushing right in, wait a minute or two to see whether he is really awake. If so, it's probably time to feed him. Very young babies normally need to eat every three hours, and in some cases every two hours.

By four or five months, night feeding is no longer necessary. Babies should be able to go without a feeding for at least a six-hour stretch. You can check him when he wakes and cries, but at this age, babies can learn to soothe themselves, rather than rely on you to pick them up or rock them. They may find their fingers. They may latch onto a pacifier or find other things in the immediate environment to interest them, such as music or a crib mobile. A flickering shadow on the ceiling or sounds outside the window may catch their attention. They might even toss and turn as adults do. They learn to distract themselves rather than depend on external aids. Babies who can learn self-soothing gain a skill that will carry them through life.

That said, of course use good sense and listen to your instincts. If a four-month-old wakes and it's been six hours since he ate, he may be hungry again. Feed him. When you've ruled out hunger, you might go in and pat his back, but try not to pick him up. If you do, the crying will probably stop, but he won't learn to settle himself. Remember, the goal is to encourage your baby's self-reliance and independence.

Is gender a factor in babies' sleep problems?

Some people think baby boys have more sleep difficulties than girls, but this isn't true. However, 61 percent of SIDS victims are male babies, for unknown reasons.

THE NEXT PHASE

When should the baby be able to sleep through the night?

There is a turning point when the baby begins to sleep through the night (i.e., at least six hours straight), and that is a very different scenario from the early days. If you're lucky, and have "a dream baby," she may start to sleep through the night at two months. More often, it takes four or five months. If you have a colicky baby who is up screaming in distress all night, the first three months can be hard going. It helps to know that colic is temporary and does end after three months. See Chapter 4 for more information on colic, plus ways to get a screaming baby to sleep.

Should I add cereal to the bottle to help my baby sleep better?

Some parents think adding cereal to the baby's bottle will speed up sleeping through the night. This is a bad idea.

Young infants do wake at night, sometimes due to hunger and sometimes due to neurological immaturity. In the latter case, stuffing them with cereal won't help them sleep any better and may contribute to obesity and acquisition of food allergies. If hunger is the problem, breastfeeding or a bottle solves it. Solids are not needed nutritionally before four to six months. In addition, cereal in a bottle clogs the nipple.

How should we transition the baby from our room to his own room?

Because lack of sleep plagues parents, I urge them to move the baby to a separate room or space at four or five months. Sleeping babies can make a great deal of noise, which is perfectly normal. You hear every coo, whimper, and start when the baby is in the same room with you, which disturbs your own sleep, not to mention your sex life. Also, when the baby sleeps outside your room, you won't be tempted to run in at every gurgle.

A sensitive noise monitor near the crib can be helpful in certain situations. For example, my daughter lives in a three-level house and uses the monitor to keep track of her baby's activity during nap time. Noise monitors are different from heart rate and respiratory monitors, which once were thought to help prevent SIDS. In fact, the latter do not prevent SIDS, and they make parents crazy because they keep going off. However, certain newborns with complex medical problems may be sent home from the hospital with a cardiac/respiratory monitor.

What if the baby still won't sleep through the night after five months?

By this time your baby should be able to sleep at least six hours straight. If this is not happening, she may be hungry because she's outgrowing her breast milk supply and is

What You Should Know about Sleep Equipment
It's fun to browse through baby stores, walking up and down the aisles checking out what's new in baby furniture and equipment, but don't confuse "new" or "pricey" with "best for baby" or practical for you. A full-size crib, which is subject to mandatory federal safety standards, is safest. (Be aware, however, that old cribs may not have been subject to those standards.)

Bassinets and cradles are other options, but these are only subject to voluntary safety standards and are quickly outgrown. For additional peace of mind, you can check bassinets and cradles for certification by the Juvenile Products Manufacturers Association (JPMA), which is based on standards set by ASTM International, the largest standards development organization in the world.

Play yards or travel yards, which are smaller than full-size cribs, come with a bassinet attached. They are subject to voluntary safety standards from the Consumer Products Safety Commission and ASTM. They are great for travel and when you're in a pinch but should not replace permanent cribs. Look for the JPMA certification seal.

Co-sleepers are separate baby beds that attach to your bed. This is the closest thing to bed sharing. Both the American Academy of Pediatrics (AAP) and *Consumer Reports* advise against using them. No safety standards are set for co-sleepers at this time.

ready for solid foods. Or she may have developed the dysfunctional sleep habits described earlier. These bad habits are not preordained. If you can, it's a lot easier to prevent them in the first place than to undo them later. If it's too late for that, you're going to have to put her down in the crib while still awake every night, and expect crying because she hasn't had any practice settling herself. If you go in to check that the problem isn't a dirty diaper or something amiss, try to be discreet. It's a challenge to tolerate crying at this stage, but try to look at the long-term goal versus short term pain. It helps to remember what I call "The Rule of Eight." Pretend you have eight children. Parents in large families don't have these problems with babies' sleep because they won't put up with them. They put the baby to bed and say, "That's it. Good night sweet love."

I want to play with the baby when I come home from work. My wife says I get him too excited, and he won't go to sleep. What should I do?

Overstimulation can impact sleep. A parent may, rightfully, want time to tickle and play with the baby after being away all day. The activity may delay bedtime, which is fine at this age. Baby may sleep better at night. Just be aware that a winding down period is important afterward in the evening. A warm bath, a feeding, and some quiet time (a book and/or lullaby) leading to sleep benefits everyone in the household.

NAPS AND OTHER SLEEPING SITUATIONS

Is it ever okay to sedate my baby to keep her from crying and to get her to sleep, for instance when we're traveling?

Some parents use cold medications to make the baby groggy, but babies should not be sedated for convenience. If your child is not a good traveler, don't travel—or leave the baby at home with Grandma or a trusted babysitter instead. Babies may cry, but cold medications can have side effects, such as seizures and respiratory depression, and should not be given to children under six years old (and then only for upper respiratory infection for those under six).

My baby only gets short naps in the car because I have to pick up my four-year-old from preschool or playdates. Is he getting enough sleep or should I ask someone else to pick up my older child?

Second and subsequent children learn to be flexible. Although a regular feeding and nap schedule is ideal, the reality of life today is that baby number two will often have to be carted around. It does balance out. What children lose in constancy, they gain in ability to adapt.

Variations in Bedtimes

There are sometimes cultural differences in baby care. A large international Internet-based survey by Jodi Mindell, PhD, Saint Joseph's University, Philadelphia, found that those differences can extend to when babies are put to sleep at night. Babies and toddlers in China, Japan, Korea, India, and nine other Asian countries went to bed later and got less total nighttime sleep than children in the United States, United Kingdom, Australia, New Zealand, and Canada. Bedtimes ranged from 7:27 p.m. in New Zealand to 10:17 p.m. in Hong Kong, with the U.S. bedtime clocking in at 8:52 p.m. Asian babies and toddlers were more likely to room share, as well, and more of their parents reported sleep problems in their children than parents in predominantly Caucasian countries.

How many naps should my baby have?

Your baby will determine this. In the first few months the nap pattern will vary from sleeping all day with brief breaks to eat—all the way to being awake most of the day with short catnaps. From six months to one year, most babies take at least two naps. They give up the second nap at some point during the second year.

My mother-in-law takes care of the baby three days a week and lets him nap too long. How can I get her to shorten naps?

It's important to give clear guidelines about sleep to caregivers when a baby is past the newborn stage. Specify the times you want naps to start and finish and don't let anyone undermine your instructions. When my own children were young, a caregiver might let the baby sleep all afternoon. That was a real problem. My husband and I insisted that afternoon naps had to start early in the afternoon and last a maximum of two hours. There's nothing worse than coming home from work at 5:00 p.m. and finding your child asleep. You think to yourself, "Now the baby will be up till midnight, and I'm just doomed."

My son slept through the night at four months. Now he's older and has started getting up in the middle of the night. Why is this happening?

This pattern is actually very typical. Sometimes between six and nine months the baby suddenly wakes up at night. Parents often explain it away with, "Oh, he's teething," because that's what someone else said to them. Actually, the cause may be developmental change. For example, a baby might roll over, which he's never done before, and wake himself up. Or he might stand up in the crib and be unable to get back down again by himself. He's stuck, so he cries. And sometimes babies wake up at night just as adults do. When babies wake under these circumstances, they experience separation anxiety and start fussing. They want to know where you are.

If the baby keeps crying, check to make sure he isn't sick (without picking him up). Did he vomit or does he have a fever? Feel his head to see if it's warm. Look for a wet or dirty diaper. If that's the problem, you do have to change the diaper to prevent a rash. Otherwise, let him learn to set-tle back to sleep on his own. I know this is hard to do, but it's best. I remember one mom who sheepishly confided to me that she was so anxious to get her nine-month-old back to sleep that she crawled into the crib with him and curled into a ball until he dozed off. This is not a helpful solution.

What clothing should the baby sleep in?

Choose comfortable, roomy clothes that do not bind. In warm weather a diaper and undershirt are fine, or a light one-piece "onesie." In winter a warm undershirt, diaper, and blanket sleeper with feet do the job. You can always add a layer of clothing when it's cold.

Do babies dream?

Research says they do. REM (rapid eye movement) sleep, which was first discovered in 1953, is the period of sleep when dreams occur. Research back in the 1960s observed REM sleep in newborns. Half of their sleep time is REM sleep versus 20 percent to 25 percent for adults.

SIDS FACTS

How prevalent is SIDS and what causes it?

Most new parents tend to obsess about SIDS because they feel helpless to prevent it. As horrifying as the thought of SIDS may be, the incidence is very small—0.01 percent. There are many possible causes of SIDS such as infection, immature respiratory center (an area of the brain that regulates breathing), cardiac arrhythmia, and suffocation (both accidental and intentional).

Are there cultural differences in susceptibility to SIDS?

The SIDS risk for African American babies is more than double the risk for Caucasian babies. American Indian and

Native Alaskan infants have triple the risk. Premature babies from any culture are at higher risk than full-term infants.

I've heard that it's a good idea to give my baby a pacifier when she's put to sleep. Why? I'd rather not use a pacifier.

Historically pediatricians have been taught that pacifier use in newborns may lead to nipple confusion when nursing, sloppy speech patterns, dental malocclusion, and other problems. However, research has shown a significant reduction in the risk of SIDS when babies go to sleep with a pacifier. In 2005 the American Academy of Pediatrics revised its recommendations to include pacifier use in infants as a means of preventing SIDS.

Offer a pacifier any time you put the baby down to sleep, including naps. (Because it takes time for an infant to become accustomed to breastfeeding, postpone a pacifier for breastfed babies until the child is nursing well.) Some infants will resist a pacifier at first and may have to be taught to accept it. Keep trying gently and eventually most infants will learn to latch on.

You can try to wean from the pacifier at around nine months, but I don't recommend it any earlier. Although SIDS risk is highest in the first three or four months, SIDS can occur any time in the first year. The research on pacifiers and reduction of SIDS risk did not address when it is safe to wean pacifiers.

Why is it important for babies to sleep on their backs?

In 1992 the AAP recommended that infants sleep on their backs rather than in a prone (face down) position and launched a "Back to Sleep" public awareness campaign. Since then the SIDS rate has declined dramatically. Most American infants now sleep on their backs. Putting the baby down to sleep on its side is not a safe option because the child may roll over onto the stomach. Older babies may find their own way to the side-sleeping position, but there's not much you can do about it. Once they're able to roll over, they're strong enough to lift their heads and thus resist accidental suffocation—one of the main hazards of sleeping on the stomach.

Cutting SIDS Risk

There are steps you can take to help protect your baby from SIDS, starting with room sharing for the first four or five months (although it's fine to nurse or cuddle the baby in your bed). Always put the baby to sleep on his back and offer a pacifier. Take these crib precautions:

- Use a firm mattress
- No bumpers
- No loose blankets, quilts, pillows in the crib
- No stuffed animals or other toys in the crib
- In addition, dress your baby lightly for sleep if it's warm, or in layers topped by a blanket sleeper with feet if it's cold. Make your household a smoke-free environment.

A mother's smoking during pregnancy is a risk factor for SIDS, and environmental smoke has been linked to increased incidence of SIDS. One study found using a fan during sleep resulted in a 72 percent reduction in SIDS.

Should I still put the baby to sleep on her back when she has a cold? Should I sleep in her room until the cold improves?

Your baby should always be put to sleep on her back, but she may be more comfortable sleeping slightly upright while battling a cold. Many parents feel more secure sleeping close to the baby for the duration of a cold or other illness, but it's a judgment call.

My friend's baby has flat spots on his head from sleeping on his back. How can I prevent that?

A phenomenon called positional plagiocephaly has become more of an issue since babies have been switched to sleeping on their backs. The condition is characterized by flat spots or bald areas on the head, and occurs because infants do tend to lay down their heads favoring one side or the other. These spots are correctable with time once the baby is old enough to roll over and no longer lie in the same head position for extended periods (at around four to five months old). I encourage parents to give babies supervised tummy time to get them off their head and strengthen their upper bodies. If the baby always looks to the left and is getting a spot, position her so that all the activity in the room is on the right. This will encourage her to turn her head. Reverse it if the baby always looks to the right.

MORE FEARS

Sometimes I listen to my newborn breathing while she's sleeping, and she seems to take a long pause before catching her breath. Is this normal? I'm afraid she's stopped breathing.

What you describe is called periodic breathing, where a newborn takes several short breaths followed by a pause. This is perfectly normal. She should outgrow periodic breathing in a few weeks. If not, tell your doctor.

What if the baby spits up while sleeping? Could he choke?

Babies can spit up during sleep, but they're unlikely to choke. If your child spits up frequently, consider elevating the mattress slightly to raise his head higher than his feet. However, this will not work if a baby is old enough to move around in the crib.

Talking Together

Sit down with your partner and say, "Let's talk about how the baby will fall asleep, and what we'll do when she wakes up crying." Many parents cannot tolerate crying or fussing and regularly pick up an older baby to stop the noise. They think giving in is a short-term solution. It is not, and only makes it more difficult for the baby to sleep through the night. This issue can be a lightning rod for parental stress and cause a lot of tension between you if one partner is a soft touch and feels it's really mean to let a baby cry. I see many couples at odds. Often at the sixth-month visit, the husband complains to me, "We get no sleep. Every time the baby whimpers, she picks him up and feeds him. I'm so tired in the morning, I drag myself to the office. I think the baby is perfectly able to sleep through the night without nursing, if she'd just leave him alone."

Typically, the baby is still sleeping in the parents' room. Mom hears him fussing, and it is easier for her to feed him than to ignore his whimpers. The baby is enjoying two wonderful but probably unnecessary meals each night at two and four in the morning, and he has mom's undivided attention. Dad's reaction is another matter.

When you and your spouse disagree on this or any other matter, and many times it is the father who is the soft touch, the situation is best resolved in the light of day before exhaustion, a screaming baby, sleep deprivation, and hormones cloud the discussion. One answer may be to make your pediatrician the final arbiter. In instances like the one above, I reassure the mom that the baby doesn't need a feeding for at least six hours—and will make up any lost calories when feeding during the day. The most important consideration is that the baby learns to self-soothe at this age.

BE PROACTIVE

Like the rest of us, babies are creatures of habit. Whatever practices you employ to get your baby to sleep will quickly become a pattern. A simple, loving action such as regularly rocking your infant to sleep may seem natural and soothing for both parent and child, but what is a bonding experience at two weeks may seem like a noose at six months. You and your partner can avoid such traps by planning together.

Now that there's a baby in the household, this is also a time to examine the role alcohol plays with your family—and your own drinking habits. If you're accustomed to having a few drinks in the evening, realize that alcohol is a sedative, and you need to be up and alert at night—ready to go from zero to ten—as a parent.

Realize, too, that parenting a baby is not an exact science, and guidelines are just that—guidelines. They can change as new information comes to light and as circumstances we never imagined arise in this complex world. Trust your judgment, be flexible, and talk to your pediatrician when in doubt. Then everyone will get a good night's sleep.

CHAPTER 2

Breastfeeding—
Issues and Challenges

This chapter covers:
- Getting started
- Breastfeeding problems and solutions
- Mothers' medications and the effects on babies
- Pumping and storing breast milk
- Weaning
- Formula facts

Breast milk is the ideal food for babies, and most babies born in the United States are breastfed at least initially. Because the benefits are so significant, a push is underway to increase the numbers and to encourage mothers to breastfeed for a longer period of time than most currently do. Breastfeeding is good for your baby, good for you, and so much more convenient than formula. It can take time to establish breastfeeding because both you and the infant are on a learning curve. The key to success is patience, persistence, and support when you need it.

Parents typically ask me these questions about breastfeeding:

BEGINNER BASICS

What are the advantages of breastfeeding?
Breast milk is easier for babies to digest than formula and also offers the perfect mix of nutrients and vitamins for healthy growth and development. Breast milk builds babies' immune systems, and there seems to be a lower incidence

of obesity in breastfed babies. In the first year of life, I find these babies are definitely slimmer. There is also some protection from SIDS , which may be due to antibodies in breast milk.

Once breastfeeding is established, the experience itself can be a source of relaxation and connection with your baby. The skin-to-skin contact promotes maternal bonding, and many mothers cherish this special time together. We now know that the sooner you start breastfeeding the better. The baby should be put to the breast right after birth.

Breastfeeding also helps you regain your pre-pregnancy shape faster because it burns about 500 calories a day. Certain hormonal effects from breastfeeding speed your body's recovery from giving birth by contracting the uterus. Breastfeeding also reduces your risk for breast and ovarian cancer.

How does breastfeeding protect my baby from illness?

Some antibodies in mothers' milk are protective against certain illnesses. For example, research suggests breastfed babies may get fewer ear infections and be less susceptible to diarrhea and some respiratory problems. But you have antibodies only if you've had the particular variety of virus— and viruses mutate all the time. This means your baby is still vulnerable to some infection, which is why you should take normal precautions. Wash your hands after changing a diaper and ideally before handling your baby. For the first eight weeks, encourage hand washing before anyone touches the baby. It may sound overcautious, but that's one way viruses are transmitted.

Don't let sick people, such as someone with a bad cold, touch the baby. Avoid exposing the baby to crowds at least for the first two months.

Do I have to breastfeed?

Breastfeeding is the best way to feed your baby. Today, there's a lot of support in hospitals including postpartum nurses trained in lactation, nursery physician support, and lactation specialists to help you and the baby get off to a good start. However, breastfeeding doesn't work for all women. Some have inverted nipples that make it difficult for the baby to latch on to the breast. With help, these mothers can breastfeed. Or they may have breast augmentation that can interfere with developing a good milk supply. I've counseled women who feel uncomfortable breastfeeding, or who can't relax and wind up obsessing about whether the baby is getting enough milk.

Some women are not able to breastfeed for medical reasons. For example, HIV-positive mothers can transmit the infection to the baby through breast milk, and in the United States they are told they should not breastfeed. (However, some developing countries have different recommendations.) Mothers who must take certain medications that pass into breast milk and have the potential to harm the baby should also refrain from breastfeeding.

If there are reasons not to breastfeed, you can find a pediatrician who will support you. Do not feel guilty if you can't (or decide not to) do it. There are plenty of healthy formula-fed babies, and there are situations where breastfeeding is not optimal for the mother or the child. But if possible, give breastfeeding a try and get all the help you need from a lactation consultant and/or your pediatrician, who may have special training in lactation issues.

How often should I breastfeed?

Most people do demand feeding, which usually amounts to eight to twelve times in twenty-four hours, although it can be more often. Frequent feeding stimulates production of breast milk, which comes in at around three to five days after the birth of your child. When breast milk is in, I advise mothers to breastfeed no more than once every two hours. This is important because sometimes a baby will use you as a pacifier. The average feeding on one breast can take any-where from seven-and-a-half to twenty minutes, depending on how the baby sucks, milk flow, and other factors. If feed-ing time is slower, that's fine, but it should not take more than forty minutes. Otherwise, your nipples can get very raw and irritated, and even start to bleed. If this happens, once the baby is a month old and accustomed to breast-feeding, you can offer a pacifier if she wants to suck longer. Breastfeeding is meant to be a pleasurable experience for you and your baby, not an ordeal.

There is another reason to generally limit demand feeding to once every two hours. Babies who constantly feed will develop the tendency to suck and graze all day long, which does not allow the still-delicate intestinal tract to rest. Occasionally, of course, there will be times when you do feed more often. But you don't want to become exhausted and feel trapped. Too often a mother will com-plain to me, "All I do is feed." Within the first few weeks the baby should get into the rhythm of feedings every two or three hours.

Should I wake up my baby to feed?

Babies lose weight while in the hospital because they're born with extra body fluid that is excreted in the first few days after birth. If your newborn has lost more than 10 per-cent of birth weight when discharged from the hospital, your pediatrician may tell you to wake and feed her to sup-ply necessary nutrition until the weight is regained (usually by ten days of age), Once the weight issue is resolved, you can let her sleep longer at night—four or five hours—without nursing. Daytime is different. I advise waking up the baby to feed during the day if she sleeps more than three hours straight. Otherwise babies can mix up night and day. They sleep all day and are up all night.

I have small breasts. Will that affect breast milk production?

Small glands in the breast produce milk, and the baby's sucking stimulates milk production. Breast size has nothing to do with milk supply.

Does my baby need anything besides breast milk until he starts solids?

Breast milk is truly a complete food for babies. However, current research shows Vitamin D, which is essential for building bones, may have to be added because breast milk does not contain enough of it. This is true especially if you live at a latitude (such as the Northeast) where the baby's exposure to sunlight may be limited. Ask your pediatrician whether a Vitamin D supplement is necessary in your baby's case.

Does breastfeeding help babies sleep through the night sooner?

My experience has been that bottle-fed babies are actually the ones who sleep through the night faster. But breastfeeding has a long list of other important advantages. You can't have everything.

COMMON PROBLEMS

What should I do if my baby refuses to take the breast?

This can happen when you start breastfeeding for any number of reasons. Sometimes your areola, the area surrounding the nipple, and the nipple itself are too big if you're engorged. Or the baby may be too sleepy after delivery to be interested in feeding at all. Or he's frustrated because your milk has not come in. He may not have mastered the ability to latch onto your breast successfully. If so, you can talk to your pediatrician or lactation consultant about ways to show the baby how to latch on properly. Also try to feed the baby as soon as you see he's hungry. If you wait too long and he works up to a screaming rage, he'll get so aggravated that he won't latch on. You know your baby wants to feed if he starts stirring and makes sucking sounds.

In general, loss of appetite can be a sign of illness in a baby. If you think your child is sick, call the doctor. When an older baby refuses the breast, it may be due to thrush, a fungal infection in the oral mucous membrane.

What are inverted nipples, and what can you do about them?

Inverted nipples turn in rather than out. They are common and are not abnormal, but they can make it harder for a baby to latch on and feed. If you're having trouble, consult your lactation specialist or your pediatrician for help.

What causes bleeding nipples, and what can I do about this?

Nipples start bleeding because the baby is not latching on to the nipple properly or is sucking too long. Your obstetrician can give you one of several creams to help reduce irritation. It is also helpful to expose your breast to the air to dry after feeding.

I've noticed a rash on my breasts. Does it have anything to do with breastfeeding?

Yeast is frequently found on the skin as part of normal flora along with bacteria. Yeast can multiply and cause a skin infection, especially in a warm and moist area. A suckling infant can create the perfect environment for a yeast infection on your breasts. If you have this infection, you may transmit the yeast to the baby's mouth, causing thrush. A baby-safe antifungal cream prescribed by your obstetrician can clear up the skin infection. Similarly, your baby's pediatrician can prescribe an antifungal medication to treat thrush inside the baby's mouth.

My baby bites my breasts and it hurts. Is there a way to stop this?

The biting is not intentional, but it is painful. Once your baby gets teeth, she may find it soothing to use your nipple as a teething ring. When this occurs, remove your nipple from her mouth. Then resume breastfeeding, making sure the baby is fully latched on. It helps to give her a teething ring—frozen teething rings work well—for the chewing she needs to do.

Should I supplement with formula until my breast milk comes in?

You usually don't have to. But if the baby has significant jaundice, which turns the skin (and often the whites of the eyes) yellow—or is dehydrated or has lost more than 10 percent of his birth weight on discharge from the hospital—he may need a day or two of formula until breast milk comes in at around day four. This is a judgment call your pediatrician will help you make. Occasionally some babies must be hospitalized because they didn't receive the supplementation they needed.

My baby has turned yellow after several weeks of breastfeeding. Why?

The baby may have breast milk jaundice, which affects roughly 2 percent of newborns. When breast milk jaundice occurs, the liver is temporarily inhibited from processing a chemical in the body called bilirubin. The baby looks yellow as a result. Breast milk jaundice is easily cured when breast feeding is stopped for twenty-four hours. We don't know why. The problem just clears up. The diagnosis should be made by your pediatrician because there are other causes of jaundice in an infant, such as bile blockage, hepatitis, or certain anemias, although these are rare. A blood test will probably be done to confirm an elevated bilirubin and to rule out other problems if jaundice persists.

My breasts keep leaking. What should I do?

You can buy nursing pads from the drug store to wear inside your bra to absorb leaked milk.

Can a baby be allergic to breast milk?

Dairy products in your own diet transmit cow's milk protein to your baby in your breast milk. Some babies are allergic to cow's milk protein (which is also contained in formula). A sign of the allergy is blood in the baby's stool, especially if accompanied by mucus, and sometimes gas and colicky behavior.

A usual treatment is to stop eating dairy yourself—and possibly abstain from soy, because often babies allergic to cow's milk protein are also allergic to soy. A formula-fed baby who is allergic will be switched to an elemental formula (i.e., one that does not contain cow's milk protein). See Chapter 12 for additional information on allergies. If bleeding in the stool continues despite these changes, your pediatrician will probably refer the baby to a gastroenterologist to check out other possible causes.

How long should I breastfeed?

The AAP recommends that babies breastfeed exclusively for at least the first six months—and, ideally for the first year. Those are important goals. At present, however, only 13.6 percent of babies are still being exclusively breastfed

Medications and Breastfeeding

Medications have the potential to get into your breast milk and to affect the baby or interfere with milk production. Even if they were safe during your pregnancy, breastfeeding is different. That's why it's essential if you are nursing to check with your pediatrician before taking any over-the-counter or prescription drug. Some medications are acceptable, such as ibuprofen or acetaminophen for pain, penicillin for infections, insulin for diabetes, and certain drugs for allergies, cardiovascular problems, depression, asthma, and other conditions. Often there is an alternative medication you can use if a drug is off limits. In certain situations, timing can make a difference, such as taking a drug after breastfeeding rather than before. In general, play it safe and don't take a medication unless you really need it.

We often don't think of alcohol as a drug, but it is one—and it reduces milk production. If you want to have a drink, limit your intake to a single five-ounce glass of wine, twelve ounces of beer, or one-and-a-half ounces of eighty-proof liquor per day. And wait two hours after drinking to breastfeed. As for caffeine, the AAP recommends moderation—two or three cups of caffeinated drinks, including coffee, a day. If you smoke cigarettes, you're putting your baby in double jeopardy. There's a risk of nicotine getting into the milk supply, plus the danger of secondhand smoke.

without any formula supplementation by six months. There are many reasons for the drop off. Many women go back to work after maternity leave, and may find breast pumping hurdles on the job too difficult. Others who stay home may resume hectic pre-baby lives. It can just seem more practical to be able to mix up a bottle of formula, at least at times, rather than pump breast milk. Many women combine breast milk and formula feeding.

If you introduce a bottle after a few weeks of breast-feeding, your baby is more likely to take a bottle. You can use pumped breast milk in the bottle instead of formula, which allows dad and others to feed the baby.

The longer you breastfeed, the better it is for your baby. Yet some employers are more breastfeeding-friendly than others. Some jobs are more demanding than others. Only you can make the decision in view of your personal circumstances.

PUMPING AND STORING BREAST MILK

When should I start pumping breast milk?

Once your milk supply is well established (after a couple of weeks), you can start using a breast pump to draw milk for use when you can't be there in person at feeding time, such as when you're at work, have a babysitter, or your spouse is going to give a feeding.

Try to pump two or three times over an eight-hour period—for ten to fifteen minutes each time. Always pump after you've fed the baby to avoid diminishing the milk supply before feeding.

What kind of pump should I buy?

A wide variety of breast pumps are available today. You can choose from manual and electrical models in different weights and sizes and with different features at prices ranging from about $35 to $1,000 or more for certain hospital-grade pumps. You may also wish to consider renting a pump. The length of time you plan to use the pump can help you decide whether the rental option will work for you. Consumer Reports reviews pump models and offers recommendations. You can check it online to help you make the best choice for your situation and price range. Some of this information is free online, although you must subscribe to get a complete report. If you don't subscribe, perhaps a friend does and can check it for you, or the magazine may be available at the library.

How long can I store breast milk?

You can keep breast milk at a room temperature of up to 77 degrees for up to eight hours. The milk can be stored for up to five days in the back of the refrigerator, and in a refrigerator's separate freezer (with a separate door) for three to six months.

How do I wean the baby?

More than half of mothers of babies less than a year old in the United States are employed. If you're weaning to bottle feed with breast milk because you're returning to work or for other reasons, you can introduce the bottle after breastfeeding is firmly established. The challenge is to get the baby used to the bottle and a different nipple. Many babies will not take a bottle if you wait too long. It is also easier to have dad or someone else offer the bottle. Babies are smart, and if they know "the real thing" is available, they may hold out. Mothers often can't successfully introduce the bottle because the baby smells the milk in their breasts.

Many mothers are able to go back to work and pump on site. Some lactation-friendly employers, especially large ones, provide a special room for this purpose. For other moms, the hurdles involved may make pumping on the job difficult or impossible. If necessary, do both breastfeeding and formula. Many mothers breastfeed in the morning and at night and formula feed when the child is at day care or home with a nanny or sitter. Some babies take formula readily from a bottle. If the baby does not accept it easily, just slowly mix in the formula with breast milk until the baby gradually accepts it.

On the other hand, if you breastfeed exclusively for a long period, at about six months of age you can skip the bottle step and begin introducing pumped breast milk in a "sippy cup." You'll hold this cup, which comes with a cover and nipple to prevent spills. Be aware that the baby will take a lot less breast milk in the cup than he did when breastfeeding. That's fine, as long as he continues to urinate every four hours or so. At this age you want him to eat solids rather than fill up on breast milk. The sooner you wean your baby to a cup, the easier it is, which is why this should ideally be done between eight or nine months and one year.

History Lesson

Breastfeeding your baby dates back to primitive times, when mother's milk was the only nourishment available. The popularity of breastfeeding has fluctuated throughout history, however. For example, for centuries many wealthy women used wet nurses to breastfeed for them because nursing was considered undignified and "beneath them." It was lower class women who fed their own babies. Families in Western Europe often farmed out their infants to wet nurses in rural areas.

Wet nursing was imported to the United States when European settlers arrived—and faded in the early twentieth century. In the 1950s, most babies were bottle fed. Today, scientific knowledge of the benefits of breastfeeding has made it the preferred way to nourish babies.

FORMULA

If I use formula for partial or total feeding, what is the best formula to buy?

Several brands are easily available in supermarkets and drug stores. I usually recommend choosing a formula fortified with iron (to build red blood cells), and with added lipids and fatty acids to make it similar to breast milk. These fatty acids are thought to aid vision and brain development. Formula is available in powder, liquid concentrate, and ready to feed form.

How should I prepare formula?

Follow the directions on the label. The Food and Drug Administration (FDA) advises sterilizing bottles and nipples in the dishwasher or in boiling water for five minutes. Once the baby starts to put things in his mouth (around three months) and is past the dangerous stage for infections, you can hand wash bottles and nipples with soap and water.

How should I store formula?

Formula should be refrigerated as soon as it's mixed or opened. Use it within two days.

Can formula be reused if my baby doesn't finish the bottle?

No. Throw it out because bacteria from the baby's mouth can grow in the remaining formula. The FDA maintains a toll-free hotline—888-SAFE FOOD (733-3663)—for any questions you have on proper handling or storing of any liquid or solid food babies eat.

How should I warm formula?

You can run hot tap water over the bottle of formula for a minute or two or put the bottle in a pan of heated water (after the pan is removed from the stove). You don't want to burn the baby's mouth, so try a drop of formula on the top of your hand first. It should feel lukewarm, not hot. Do not heat bottles of formula in the microwave, due to uneven heating that can cause hot spots that can hurt the baby. Note that there is no medical reason for warming a baby's formula other than trying to mimic the human body temperature of breast milk. On a hot day, the baby might enjoy a slightly cooler drink.

Is it really necessary to stop using plastic baby bottles?

There have been health alerts about the possible danger of the chemical bisphenol A (BPA) in various products including plastic baby bottles. The concern is BPA's effect on the brain and other health issues. Current recommendations are to use BPA-free bottles, which are readily available in stores. And of course keep abreast of any new recommendations down the road.

Why do I feel like a failure because I can't breastfeed?

One of the unintended consequences in the push to convince more mothers to breastfeed is the guilt felt by women who can't (or choose not to) breastfeed. For a variety of reasons breastfeeding doesn't work out for some moms. What's most important is that you have a loving, stress-free relationship with your child and that the baby gets adequate nutrition.

Guilt doesn't do anyone any good. Nourishment can be delivered in several different ways if necessary, and babies can be fed very well with formula. Or your doctor can write a prescription for breast milk from a human milk bank, where milk is donated by lactating women. In cases of multiple births, a mother may lack enough milk to feed more than one baby.

Talking Together

Breastfeeding is not just a women's issue. Due to its nature and the time involved in getting it right, breastfeeding can raise the level of stress in the household and cause friction between spouses. It's important that both of you discuss your feelings and concerns to head off unnecessary tensions. Once anxieties are out on the table, you can start working together to problem solve.

For example, a common situation occurs if the baby doesn't get enough breast milk in the early days, before the mother's milk supply comes in fully. Babies often scream because they're still hungry, and mothers feel inadequate. Some fathers become frustrated that mom won't just go to "Plan B" and use formula. They don't understand the mother's desire to succeed at breastfeeding, and that using a bottle of formula may impede the baby's adjustment to the breast. Many times, I've seen a dynamic where the mother feels she's failed, and the father, who wants to use formula, complains, "We're not feeding the baby."

In cases where breastfeeding is difficult, it's important to seek support from your pediatrician, and possibly use a lactation consultant. I encourage continuation of breastfeeding, but also following up with a bottle of formula afterward—at least for the first few days until the milk comes in. This takes care of the screaming baby, removes the worry that he's starving, and does not interfere with establishing breastfeeding. The most important goal is to get off to a good start with the baby and provide adequate nutrition.

Sometimes a father is not supportive of breastfeeding for other reasons. Breastfeeding is a special experience between mother and baby, one that may stir jealousy in the father—or he may feel left out. There are several ways to reassure him and draw him into the circle of love. Get him involved in bonding with and nurturing the baby through other activities, such as holding and talking to her or dressing her. Dad can also feed a bottle of pumped breast milk, once breastfeeding is established. Perhaps he can take charge of bath time, where play together is natural, and take the baby to the park on Saturday while you get a manicure. Look for opportunities to tell your spouse he's needed and praise him for what he's doing right. Of course changing diapers is an equal opportunity chore.

To rally support, you can also talk about the advantages of breastfeeding that are most likely to get his attention, such as the economics—breast milk is free—and the fact that breastfeeding is a kind of contraceptive. Because breastfeeding delays menstruation, it can help you space pregnancies naturally. But don't count on breastfeeding alone. I know of breastfeeding mothers who have conceived.

SKILL BUILDING FOR YOU AND YOUR BABY

Most women breastfeed today and I encourage you to try. Be aware that nursing is a skill that takes time to master; many mothers need help and emotional support. Your partner in breastfeeding—your baby, who until now has passively been getting all his needs met in the womb—also must learn how to take the breast efficiently.

Be patient and kind to yourself as you practice together with your baby. And remember that all kinds of assistance are available to help you breastfeed successfully, including the experts at www.womenshealth.gov or 1-800-994-9662.

CHAPTER 3

Food and Nutrition— Starting Off Right

This chapter covers:

- Introducing solid foods
- Homemade baby foods
- Organic foods
- Transitioning to table foods
- Fluids: water and juices
- Concerns about obesity
- Eating with baby and the tradition of family meals
- Parents' quiz

With the food pyramid inverting itself and frightening food alerts adding to the confusion, it isn't easy to be a nutrition-conscious parent today. If you feel that feeding your baby has become fraught with emotion, expectation, and politics, you have good reason. We know that unhealthy eating at the start can put children at risk for obesity, heart disease, diabetes, and other serious health problems. You want to make sure your baby gets the vitamins and nutrients necessary for growth and develops good eating habits. Here are questions and answers that will help you reach this goal.

SOLID FOODS

When should I introduce solids?

You can start offering pureed foods to your baby somewhere between four to six months of age. By this time, babies have developed enough to be able to swallow and digest foods other than breast milk or formula, and they begin to need the iron available in iron-fortified baby cereals. They are at lower risk for allergies because their immune systems have matured. Big babies have begun to outgrow the mother's milk supply and need more nutrition. At this age babies are also old enough to sit upright in your lap or an infant seat.

Transitioning to pureed foods is an important milestone. You know your baby is ready for it when she begins to grab at the sandwich you're nibbling or stares at the mashed potatoes on your plate. Your pediatrician will help you decide when to begin this next step.

What food should I introduce first?

Most parents start with a single baby cereal, such as rice cereal, which is fortified with extra iron. Initially mix one to two teaspoons of cereal with breast milk or formula, just enough to make the mixture liquid enough to be swallowed easily. (Avoid mixing cereal or other solids in the bottle, which will clog the nipple.) Feed cereal and other solids with a small spoon—and only with a spoon—to encourage the baby to become accustomed to eating that way. Eventually she'll start trying to feed herself with the spoon at around twelve to fifteen months. Let her, even though initially she may wind up with more food on her face (or on the floor) than in her mouth.

Take it easy and slow, offering a fraction of a spoonful at first. Follow with the breast or a bottle to wash it down, which will encourage her to naturally swallow the cereal. If she tends to be constipated, try oatmeal or barley baby cereal instead of rice cereal, which is binding, and avoid bananas or applesauce when she progresses to other solids.

Why is cereal usually introduced first?

At six to nine months, babies' iron stores (which they got from their mothers in utero) start to reach their lowest point. Iron is important for red blood cell production, and red blood cells die every 120 days. The body continually makes

new blood cells to replace the loss. Baby cereals are fortified with iron to facilitate this process and prevent anemia.

My baby refuses cereal. What should I do?

Remember that textured food is a new experience for babies
and they often don't take to solids immediately. At first they
will tend to push out solids with their tongue as a carryover
reflex from nursing, and may need to learn to take cereal.
If cereal is refused, try again the next day. It may take a
dozen tries before your baby will accept it, but eventually
she will come around. I know it can be frustrating, but try to
be patient. Never push against your baby's refusal. The goal
is to make eating a pleasure, not a battle, and a time to talk
to and interact with your child.

What foods should I continue with?

The general pattern is to add either a vegetable or fruit after
a few days to a week of trying cereal without any adverse
physical reaction. Offer the new food first, before cereal,
when he's more likely to be receptive because he's hungry.
Add one new food every few days. If there's a reaction to
the food, such as a rash, try to investigate what might have
caused the reaction and stop giving the baby that food. See
Chapter 12 for more information about dealing with food
(and other) allergies in the first year.

If I introduce fruit before a vegetable, will the baby become addicted to sugar?

Babies like sweets, just as most adults do. But there's no evidence that introducing fruit before a vegetable will encourage a sweet tooth. In other words, it doesn't really matter
which comes first. Your baby may like the sweet taste of
carrots and sweet potatoes.

When should I add meats?

Pureed meats, such as chicken, turkey, and beef, should be introduced by the time your baby is eight months old. Stick with single-food jars, rather than combinations. Combination foods contain carbohydrate fillers, which add extra starch babies don't need.

My baby doesn't like meat and spits it out. What should I do?

She may be showing discernment. Baby meats in jars don't taste very good. There are many other ways to get protein into baby; you can substitute foods such as tofu, yogurt, and other dairy products. Often babies prefer white meat like chicken or turkey over dark meat.

Do I need to heat up baby food?

You don't need to heat up baby food any more than you need to heat your own food. If you do warm up baby food, be sure to test it first to make sure it isn't too hot before feeding it to your child. On a hot summer day she might even enjoy slightly chilled food.

How often should my baby eat solids?

Initially, feed solids one to two times a day—for breakfast and/or dinner. By eight or nine months, offer solids three times a day. A typical menu might include cereal and fruit in the morning; meat and a vegetable at lunch; and maybe cereal, fruit, and vegetable (and possibly another meat) at dinner. This menu is not absolute. I encourage parents to follow their instincts and be flexible. Remember, babies also get breast milk and/or formula, which offer lots of protein, as well as other nutrients.

A bonus during this transition: Solids may help your baby sleep at night now that his neurological systems have grown more mature.

Should You Make Your Own Baby Food?

It's cheaper to make your baby's food yourself and it also allows you to broaden the menu of foods your baby tries. On the other hand, do you really have the time or want to spend it in this way? Only you can decide. If you choose to make your own:

- Puree foods thoroughly to prevent the possibility of choking.
- Use iron-fortified baby cereal as a filler to provide extra iron, rather than ordinary cereal.
- Avoid adding spices and salt to pureed meats to make them tastier. Why start a salt habit when breast milk and formula already contain some salt? Babies do not need extra spices either. Why program their taste buds?
- Fresh, homemade baby foods contain no preservatives and don't keep as long in the refrigerator as jars from the supermarket. But they can be frozen.

What should I know before buying a high chair?

A high chair makes feeding solids so much easier. Your baby can progress to a high chair when he can sit without support, usually around six to eight months. Today, new high chairs are subject only to voluntary safety standards. Look for certification by the JPMA, which tells you a model has met standards for stability and other safety and practical features. This is important because high chairs can tip over. Babies can surprise you. They can squirm or stand up or engage in other antics in a high chair that can cause accidents resulting in skull fractures, concussions, broken arms or legs, lacerations, or other injuries. Always use the safety straps.

Be aware that older high chairs may not meet today's safety standards, and you want to think twice about buying one secondhand at a yard sale or using a chair that's been standing in a relative's attic for many years. If space is a problem you might want to consider a fold-up high chair.

My baby has been turning a yellow-orange color since taking solid foods. What's going on?
He may have a condition called carotenemia, which is an excess of carotene pigment deposited in baby's skin from eating orange vegetables like sweet potatoes, squash, and carrots. There's no harm in your baby looking like a pumpkin, but you can switch to green vegetables or add some variety to eliminate the coloration.

TABLE AND FINGER FOODS

When should I start table foods?
It's important to accustom your baby to different tastes and textures for both good nutrition and healthy development. At eight or nine months, introduce soft table foods such as tiny pieces of cheese, soft pasta, banana, or anything else soft that you're eating. Give small enough pieces to avoid choking if the food is swallowed whole. Mashed potatoes or the inside of a well-baked potato (mashed first) are fine, too. See how the baby handles the first table food before moving on to another. If he gags or retches, back off. Try again in a week or so. Some babies gag initially because they're not used to denser solid food.

My baby won't transition to table foods. Why?
Many parents offer Cheerios or very small pieces of meat as the first textured foods, but some babies can't make the transition from pureed foods. This is often a sensory issue where the baby can't deal with different textures. Although

most children will eventually make this leap, some take longer than others. It's very important to keep trying. Talk to and work with your pediatrician on this problem, especially if the baby gags all the time. If there is no physical reason for the problem, the pediatrician may recommend a feeding specialist (often an occupational therapist who specializes in feeding and swallowing problems).

GOING GREEN

We're vegetarians. Can the baby be vegetarian, too?
Absolutely. I advise many vegetarian families who raise very healthy vegetarian babies. However, be sure to provide enough protein (such as beans, dairy, and soy foods like tofu) and coordinate your baby's menu closely with your pediatrician.

Should we buy organic?
According to the United States Department of Agriculture (USDA), organic meat, poultry, eggs, and dairy products come from animals that do not receive growth hormones or antibiotics. Organic fruits, vegetables, and other foods are grown without most pesticides, synthetic fertilizers, radiation, or bioengineering. Farms growing organics are inspected to ensure that they follow the rules required to meet USDA organic standards. However, organic foods cost more than conventional foods, and there is no evidence that organic foods prevent disease or health problems.

Nevertheless, some people feel safer eating organic and/or want to support environmentally friendly practices. It's a personal judgment call whether the benefits for your household outweigh extra costs. Follow your own philosophy.

FLUIDS

How much water should my baby drink?

Water flushes out the body's wastes, manages body temperature, and performs other important functions. Dehydration (which is potentially lethal) can follow when we don't ingest or retain enough water. Breast milk and formula contain a lot of water, and that's generally enough for babies. By four or five months, most babies take twenty-eight to thirty-two ounces of formula and/or breast milk every three or four hours during the day.

In unusually hot weather, you may want to offer extra water, which should be sterilized until your baby is at least three months old. After three months, sterilized water becomes pointless because babies start putting things in their mouth that expose them to germs.

You also may want to offer water once your baby begins solid foods because formula or breast milk intake may drop to twenty-four to twenty-eight ounces at that time. Understand that thirst is a normal physiological response when the body needs water. If you offer water, your baby will drink when thirsty, and refuse when not thirsty. Urine output is another good measure of whether the baby needs water. If a parent tells me, "My baby doesn't drink anything," I ask, "Does he still wet?" If he does, he's fine. But if he hasn't voided in eight hours, call the doctor.

Is fluoridated water necessary for my baby?

Fluoride, a mineral that helps prevent cavities and builds strong teeth, has been an effective weapon against dental decay. Most localities fluoridate their water. But if yours doesn't, or if you use well water, your baby may need fluoride supplementation after six months of age. Note that fluoride is also found in certain foods, such as some juices and baby foods, which can lead to "too much of a good thing."

Dentists have been seeing a condition called hyperfluorosis, which stains teeth due to too much fluoridation. Check with the pediatrician and your baby's dentist to make sure she's getting the proper amount of fluoride.

Should I offer bottled, rather than tap water?

Studies show bottled water is not any healthier than tap water. We're also learning that plastic bottles pile up, and we don't want to keep generating material that creates disposal problems. If you choose bottled water, remember to sterilize it, just like tap water, until your baby is at least three months old.

Be aware, too, that some bottled waters don't contain adequate amounts of fluoride (or in some cases, any fluoride at all). If the only water your baby drinks is bottled, he may need fluoride supplementation.

When can my baby drink juice?

Babies should not drink juice until after six months of age because juice reduces appetite, keeping blood sugar high so babies are never hungry. Many children wind up preferring to drink rather than eat, and a juice habit is hard to break. It offers little nutrition since it's mostly sugar. If you're going to offer juice, make sure your baby drinks it only from a cup. Limit intake to a maximum of four ounces a day and always offer it along with a meal or a snack.

Which kinds of juice are best?

Best is no juice. If you're going to offer it late in the first year, however, look for the words "100 percent juice" on the label, which means fructose (a sugar) has not been added. Orange juice (diluted half and half with water) is probably best because it contains extra vitamin C. Calcium-fortified orange juice may be an alternative source of calcium, along with dairy products, for babies who don't drink any milk at all once the transition is made to a cup or they're weaned from breast milk. Some don't like the taste of whole milk.

OBESITY ISSUES AND NOT EATING ENOUGH

What should I do if my baby won't eat?

No healthy child ever voluntarily starved himself. I'm a big believer in offering food and if the child doesn't want it, the meal is over. Obviously your pediatrician will be monitoring growth and weight. If either is falling off, the doctor will address it. Forcing babies to eat, or otherwise conveying the message that their eating is important to you, hands children (even babies) a controlling device they can use. Unless babies are sick, they eat when they're hungry and don't eat when they're not. Respect that, and try not to focus on food. Food is a loaded issue, and it's important to be detached about it as long as you provide proper nutrition.

How can I encourage my baby to eat vegetables?

Children shouldn't dictate a meal. But if your baby refuses veggies, try to find a happy medium. There are ways to disguise vegetables and increase their appeal. Look at cookbooks that help you make vegetables and other foods attractive to young children. Continue to try different vegetables, even if they're refused at first. At some point, the baby may take a taste and like them. Distraction (as in "Look at Daddy's new red tie") often works, too, allowing you to slip in a spoonful. My own solution when my children were babies involved saying something silly to catch their attention. When they laughed, I'd sneak in a spoon of green beans. Offer healthy choices with variety, but if the baby doesn't want to eat a food, that's it. Do not offer snacks later to make up for it.

How do I know how much food is enough?

I am not a member of the clean plate club. Healthy babies have what is called a satiety center that says "full." I tell parents to offer food as long as the child is interested. If he turns his head away or closes his mouth, you know he's had enough. Realize, too, that babies become very distractible around six months when solids are introduced. You may be trying to feed your child, but he starts smiling or flirting when someone walks into the room. Or noises outside the window may grab his attention and take the focus off of eating. If this happens regularly, you may have to consider a change of location. Try feeding him in a quiet and/or dark room where the two of you can concentrate on the meal. This rarely lasts more than a month or two.

My baby keeps eating and doesn't seem to know when to stop. What should I do?

There are some babies who don't know they're full. They don't recognize satiety. You do have to use your own judgment about what's an appropriate amount of food. If necessary, you can distract her to stop the eating. Check with your pediatrician about where the baby is on the growth chart and whether she is gaining too much weight. If she's on target, her food intake isn't a problem. Be aware, too, that appetite can vary. There are times when babies eat more and other times when they eat less.

EATING TOGETHER

Should the baby eat with us once he's in the high chair?

Yes. Even if he sits with you only part of the time, this will become an entrenched family routine. It may also make him a better eater. Babies often want to eat what you're eating, and family mealtimes are an opportunity to provide a little taste of the foods you're enjoying. In the second year, when the baby gets antsy and starts throwing food around, this may become too disruptive. At that time, the answer is to either distract him with a toy or remove him. Sometime during the second year the food games usually stop. Play it by ear.

What should I do if my baby throws food on the floor?
This is common behavior at the end of the first year. The baby can treat it like a game. It's the equivalent of a video game for a baby staring at food he's dropped on the floor. Watching you pick it up ten times is even more fun. So is smearing food in his hair. You can ignore it or feed him separately, rather than at the table with you, until this phase passes. In the second year, throwing food is probably a sign he's done. Just take him out of the high chair.

I want to leave snacks around the house for my eleven-month-old, who often doesn't eat much at meal time, to encourage him to graze and gain weight. My mother says I shouldn't. Who's right?
Parents do get worried about poor eaters, but the problem is grazing leads to constant food intake. Eating all day long is a bad habit that contributes to obesity. The growth of the snack industry is partially responsible for the grazing phenomenon. People now think that if the food contains no trans fats, it's okay. But chips and cookies are still loaded with calories. Mini sizes of snack foods are deceiving, too. Who eats only one? They add up.

A meal should be an intentional routine in an established location, rather than a mindless activity where you stuff yourself nonstop. Babies should learn that people sit down at the table and say, "Now we're eating dinner." They cut the meat, take a bite, and enjoy it, and then they put the fork down and have a conversation.

Why are family meals so important?

There is evidence of long-term positive benefits when the family sits down to eat together at least once a day and each member talks about his day. To facilitate relaxing, enjoyable mealtimes, try to turn off the land line and let voicemail take calls during meals unless there's an emergency situation going on. Turn off your cell and BlackBerry. It's not only rude to interrupt a meal to take a call, it models negative behavior that isn't appreciated in the outside world and tells your child that eating together isn't very important. Of course turn off the TV during meals. See more on limiting exposure to TV in Chapter 8.

What about offering snacks in the car or the doctor's office to keep the peace?

I think it's necessary at times—in moderation. We live in a very mobile society. Driving with a screaming baby in the car isn't even safe. I estimate that 30 to 40 percent of the babies I see in my office have something in their mouths. The reality is you may have to use snacks sometimes to keep the baby quiet. We've all done it, but don't overdo it. Be sure to offer healthy snacks, and also keep them to a minimum. Avoid setting food up as a reward for behavior. Food is for nutrition, not blackmail. Otherwise, every time your child wants food he'll just scream.

Engage your baby instead of stuffing him. I sing to my grandchildren when we're in the car, which stops them in their tracks. I don't have a good voice, but babies don't care. They love music and often join in with their own songs.

OTHER ISSUES

My mother gave the baby a taste of ice cream. Is that okay?

There's no reason for babies to have ice cream. But the world is going to be trying to give it to your child, along with lollypops and all sorts of sugary treats. As long as you can control what goes into your baby's mouth, enjoy that advantage because it soon will be out of your hands. Pick your battles and don't obsess over this issue, especially with family.

Should we eliminate sugar?

You will never eliminate sugar (or salt) entirely from your baby's diet, although many families try. But you can aim for moderation. Commercial baby foods do contain sugar and salt, but most baby food companies try to keep them to a minimum. Why create a need that could cause problems down the road? Sugar can cause dental caries and provides empty calories.

Is it okay that my baby still takes a bottle at one year old instead of using a cup or nursing?

At nine to ten months, babies need anywhere from eighteen to twenty-four ounces of milk a day. Lots of parents continue the bottle because they're afraid the baby will take less milk with a cup. He will take less, but that's okay. Just offer other dairy products such as cheese or yogurt. The downside of the bottle is babies fill up on too much milk and don't want food, which could cause an iron deficiency. The best time to take the baby off the bottle is late in the first year. This isn't easy to do because babies become addicted to the bottle and they demand it. They want what they want.

Using a cup paves the way to weaning from the bottle. Hold a plastic cup filled with breast milk or formula, and give your baby a sip. At the same time, act as a model and give him a chance to imitate what you're doing by drinking from your own cup. You do have to accept that it's going to be a mess for a while.

When can I switch to whole milk from formula?

Wait until one year of age to introduce whole milk. The consensus is breast milk and formula contain the ideal nutrients for babies and should be continued for a full year.

I know that the evening bottle can wind up harming my baby's teeth. How can I prevent that?

Both breast and cow's milk contain lactose (a sugar). This is not an issue before teeth emerge. But if your baby has teeth, putting him to sleep with sugar coating his teeth invites cavities. In some cases, teeth turn black, called milk bottle caries, possibly due to a genetic predisposition. Try to wipe down teeth with gauze after the evening meal to remove sugar and prevent decay.

Do babies need vitamins?

Current thinking is that the only babies who need vitamin supplements are those who are solely breastfed and live in a region with limited sunlight, such as the Northeast or upper Midwest. In that case, evidence shows complementary Vitamin D is necessary. The Vitamin D in breast milk is not sufficient for babies in these climates. Babies who are poor eaters may need vitamin supplementation. For picky eaters, I recommend a multivitamin with Vitamin B.

Consult your pediatrician about which vitamins are appropriate. Do not dispense them on your own or because a friend is doing it. And beware of giving your baby too much of any one vitamin, which can cause a serious condition called hypervitaminosis.

How can I make sure my baby doesn't choke on finger food?

Some foods are easy to choke on, such as frankfurters; nuts and seeds; chunks of meat (depending on size and texture); popcorn; carrots and other raw vegetables; grapes; peanut

Talking Together

Sit down and discuss what, when, and how you want to feed your baby. You might even brainstorm together about creative ways to distract her in the car in lieu of offering food. Talk about your philosophy of feeding and your upbringing. Were family meals a bonding experience—or not? One mother told me, "I grew up in a family where everyone ate when they could, and the only family meals took place on holidays. My husband and I rarely eat together either, unless we're in a restaurant." The fact is a tradition of family meals can have significant benefits. Obviously, if you're eating together and communicating thoughts and ideas, you're not watching TV. I think family meals help prevent obesity because everyone eats at mealtimes, rather than all day long. It may discourage mindless eating.

Are you going to take a moderate stand on sugar—or say "No sugar ever"? Share with your spouse how you feel about snacking or "cleaning the plate" or finishing every bottle. While you were growing up, were you constantly reminded that children were starving in Africa? Think about where you are. You live in America amid plenty, not in Africa, and the biggest problem our children face is obesity.

Were you forced to eat or drink foods because they were good for you? That may affect your attitude. Are manners important to you? Most of us learn manners at the dinner table. What's important is coming to a meeting of the minds on how to handle such issues and deciding on the examples you want to set.

butter; hard, gooey, or sticky candy; and chewing gum. The issue really isn't how many teeth your baby has; it's a function of coordination. Some babies have no teeth and are very good at gumming food; other babies with teeth gag all the time. In general, cooked fruits and veggies that are easily mashed and cottage cheese are good. Ripe bananas and very soft pasta are suitable for "gummers." My own son choked on a teething biscuit. I tell parents to use frozen teething rings instead, which are safer. My concern is that a chunk of a teething biscuit can break off. Always remain in the same room with your baby while she is eating, in case of a choking incident. See Chapter 11 for information on how to handle choking.

A friend told me that honey is dangerous for babies. What's the problem?

Honey can cause botulism in babies under a year old. The issue is babies' digestive systems can't stand up to the botulism toxin that honey may contain. Honey is probably safe after your child's first birthday.

EATING HEALTHIER AS A FAMILY

We now know that if babies don't eat healthy, they can be negatively affected later in life. We also know that a well-nourished child learns better. If you as a household try to maintain healthy eating habits, your child is more likely to follow. This is a good time to revamp those habits if necessary, especially if you're a working couple with little or no interest in cooking a nutritious meal. Try to figure out how your family can eat healthier. Perhaps think about cooking meals on weekends and freezing them for reheating when you come home tired from work.

If a nanny or family member is going to be cooking for the baby, make it very clear that you don't want salt, sugar, or spices added to the baby's food. This first year is the last time you can totally control what goes into your baby's mouth. Once children get out of the house and visit friends or go to school, they're offered junk food and other edibles of questionable value. This first year is an opportunity to plan ahead in a relaxed, thoughtful, family-centered way.

QUIZ: HOW DO YOU REALLY FEEL ABOUT FOOD?

People have all sorts of emotional issues with food. Examine yours by answering *yes* or *no* to the following statements:

1. I have had an eating disorder. _____

If you've been bulimic or anorexic, be careful not to project the same obsessions about weight on to your baby. Whatever you do, do not restrict your baby's calories, unless it's at your pediatrician's direction. Reducing food intake without medical reason is inappropriate and dangerous to a baby, as is focusing on low fat or low carbohydrate foods. These may be healthy for you, but babies need fats and carbohydrates to thrive. If you obsess that your baby is too fat, but the doctor says her weight is normal, it's wise to discuss this with a psychotherapist.

2. I always read every word on food labels. _____

Obsessing over germs and whether food for your baby is safe to eat can result in unhealthy dietary restrictions. Fears and phobias can be instilled in your child, as well. It's important to take a balanced approach toward food. We should all advocate for the healthiest food supply, but it is easy (and expensive) to go overboard.

If your answer is yes, recognize that the real issue is fear. Are you afraid of pesticides or other perceived poisons in food, such as additives, harming your baby? Are you afraid that not eating the right foods will cause cancer or osteoporosis? Some parents go to extremes.

3. If my baby is eating, I feel reassured that he's healthy.   _____

If your answer is yes, you may come from a culture where overfeeding babies is common and a fat baby signifies health. But overeating does not equal well being. It may be hard to abandon that connection, but obesity is one of the biggest health challenges we face. What is important is appetite and growth. Your pediatrician will monitor this carefully.

4. When my baby rejects food, I feel that I'm being rejected.   _____

It is common to personalize your baby's food rejection. When he spits that rice cereal or banana concoction or drops a grilled cheese sandwich on the floor, you may feel that you are doing something wrong. But sometimes babies are just not hungry. They may be distracted or they may be trying to get a reaction from you. Keep the emotion out of feeding. Parents tend to feel like failures if their children won't eat, but babies' lack of appetite has nothing to do with you. They eat what they need.

5. I am overweight.   _____

If you are overweight, it's important to discuss with your doctor whether there might be a genetic component. When other family members are also overweight, there may be a predisposition to obesity and your baby could be at risk. Just being aware of a potential problem is helpful. Much work is being done on this front to understand the relationship between obesity and genetics. Work with your pediatrician to balance the baby's food intake and physical activity. Yes, babies do need exercise in the form of floor time and the freedom to move around. Beware of regularly keeping your child in a car seat or bouncy chair for extended periods of time. Instruct caretakers to avoid this, too.

6. I come from a family that fixated on weight. _____

If your answer is yes, you may take extreme positions regarding nutrition, which can backfire. My mother never allowed candy, for example—only chewing gum. And I became a candyholic. I still eat candy every day as an adult. Don't make a big issue of any particular food because it can create the opposite effect from what you're hoping for.

7. Celebrations in my family were always centered on food. _____

Food tends to be the center of virtually all family gatherings, celebrations, and rewards in most extended families. Consider the role you want food to play in your household. Can you take an informed, thoughtful, relaxed approach? Food should be enjoyed and certainly can be the anchor of family gatherings, but be mindful that food is nourishment—not a way of life. It's a good thing to come together over family meals, but try to keep the focus on each other rather than the fare. (Have you noticed that when you're fully engaged in conversation you tend to eat less?)

8. We always have a drink every night. _____

Do you need to have a drink every night, or a bottle of wine? Have you been a binge drinker in the past? Many women have already abandoned or cut back on alcohol during pregnancy. As a parent you need to have your wits about you, and you may be sleep deprived. Being slightly impaired can be a problem if you must race the baby to the emergency room in the middle of the night.

CHAPTER 4

Crying—Breaking the Code

This chapter covers:

- Why babies cry
- Answering (and coping with) crying
- Using signing to reduce crying
- Colic and crying
- Handling frustration and stress

The sound of your baby crying can seem like that sweet taste of a cappuccino first thing in the morning—or the screech of fingernails across a blackboard. It's simply that crying is the language of babies, and when babies are unhappy or uncomfortable or want attention for other reasons, they let you know about it. The challenge is to figure out exactly what they're crying about in order to respond appropriately. It may take you days or weeks to learn this new language, but I assure you that as you and your baby get to know each other, you will begin to decipher what different cries mean. These are the questions parents ask me about crying—and answers that will help you handle common situations effectively.

BASIC TRAINING

Why do babies cry?

Babies usually cry to communicate their needs, which can cover a lot of territory. For example, an infant's wail may say he's hungry or cold or his diaper is wet, or that he's lying in an uncomfortable position. Or the problem may be that he's sick or in pain. In that case, crying will usually be accompanied by other signs, such as refusal to take the breast or bottle, fever, or skin that is mottled or unusually pale.

As your baby grows, he may also cry because he's tired or cranky—or for no reason at all. Crying is what babies do, although some cry more than others. Personality and temperament count. Some infants are mellow and adapt easily. Others are less flexible and have difficulty adjusting to the world outside the womb.

What should I do when my newborn cries?

The first two weeks of life are a period of becoming acquainted. Learning what your baby's cries mean is not a pure science, and most parents quickly learn to differentiate one cry from another. A blood curdling shriek can indicate pain or a threatening toddler sibling. A moan or high-pitched cry may suggest illness. In other cases, tone or intensity may signal something else, and you're faced with a process of elimination.

Has the baby just had a feeding? She may be crying because a burp didn't come up. Try gently patting her back as you hold her, which will bring up trapped air or move it along. Or put her on your lap face down and then rub her back to move air around. It's another way to get the bubble up.

Or perhaps she needs a feeding. In that case, gently massage her back to calm her down before you begin nursing. She will feed a lot better if she isn't in a screaming rage.

Check her diaper, and if that isn't the problem, touch her skin to see whether she is too hot or too cold. Is something sticking her, such as a rattle or car keys lying beneath her on the rug. Or is there a bright light shining in her eyes? If none of those possibilities is causing the tears, maybe she wants some cuddling. Physical contact with mom and dad is very important to newborns because they've spent ten months in a nice warm environment in utero, feeling the mother's heartbeat, and the warmth of the amniotic fluid. Now they're suddenly thrown out into the world, and need the security of being touched, held, snuggled, and talked to. Babies are soothed by the sound of the human voice, which is one reason why talking and singing to your child are very important. It's part of the bonding experience. You can't cuddle a newborn too much, and a soft infant carrier, where the baby faces and hugs your chest, can be helpful in minimizing crying and fussing in the early months. Just be sure the baby can breathe.

If you've fed and changed your baby and checked everything else, she just may be tired. The best thing to do to get her to sleep is rub her back, then put her down in the crib on her back, and try to settle her down before she dozes off.

As your baby gets older, she will stay awake for longer and longer periods. At around one or two months, she'll start to show interest in the environment—a shadow on the wall or a sound in the hall. But then she'll get bored and want attention. To get it, she may cry.

Can you spoil a baby?

An Australian study found that one out five new parents (and 30 percent of veteran parents) felt conflicted about picking up their crying baby. One out of four new parents thought this would spoil the baby. Uncertainty about the right response to cries increased parental stress. You may feel torn about picking up the baby, too. If so, try to relax. You can't spoil young babies. If they cry they need something, and you should address it. It is important to respond to your child's crying in the very early months to establish trust.

Babies are totally helpless and dependent, and those who become damaged in orphanages often have had no one to answer their cries. There are only two times not to respond. The first is if your baby has colic (which involves crying constantly for endless hours), both you and the baby are exhausted, and you know you've done everything you could for her. (See pages 61–65 for details on colic.)

The second time to ignore crying is when you're trying to teach your baby to self-soothe to pave the way for sleeping through the night (at about five months). If the doctor has assured you she is ready for this training, and you've checked for a wet diaper and other possible causes of distress, you know the baby's needs have been met. Because you've established trust earlier, she knows that any other time you will be there for her.

My baby didn't cry much in the hospital, but he cried all night the first night home. Why?

That's to be expected. Because hospitals send newborns home so quickly these days, some infants are still tired from the birth experience, especially first children who have been through a long vaginal delivery. You may have a false sense that you've been blessed with a low maintenance baby because he's very sleepy and doesn't cry much. But as he starts to wake up, there is often a period of adaptation when he wails. The first two weeks can be very rocky as everyone is adjusting, and often the mother's milk doesn't come in until day four or five. The baby loses weight, becomes very hungry, and of course cries. This is his only way to tell you, "I'm starving. Feed me."

The current AAP recommendation is that a physician see the baby within twenty-four to forty-eight hours from discharge. At that time, occasionally babies who have lost more than 10 percent of their weight may need supplementation with formula to tide them over until the mother's breast milk is in. If they have lost this much weight, I personally tell parents to use formula for a few days and to stop when the breast milk comes in. However, pediatricians differ about the use of extra fluids in this situation.

Is it okay to use a pacifier to stop the baby from crying?

I like pacifiers because babies do need to suck, and they use the breast as a pacifier if they don't have an alternative.

After a few weeks of this, I see mothers with raw, bleeding nipples. They're in agony every time their babies nurse. Data also suggests that offering a pacifier when the baby naps or goes to sleep for the night reduces risk of SIDS.

Why do some babies have mellow cries and others unbearable shrieks?

It's just the nature of babies. You can tell in the hospital nursery right after birth that some newborns have very relaxed cries and others sharp screeches. There are variations, just as there are with adult voices.

My three-month-old often gets cranky and tired around 4:00 p.m. and starts crying. What can I do?

One grandfather I know calls it "the sundowner effect." He experienced the phenomenon when babysitting for his grandson and got excellent results by carrying him around and singing Broadway tunes to him. Babies do love singing, whether it's a lullaby or the score of *Gypsy*. They often have prolonged crying jags in the evening when the household is humming with activity and the family stress level may be high. They may be reflecting household tension and bustle by crying or may be unwinding themselves.

I can't stand my baby's crying. What can I do?

We're all different in what we can tolerate. Some parents feel guilty, mean, and heartless if they allow their baby to cry. Some can't stand crying ever. Others understand there's a time and a place for crying—and a point where the baby is old enough to learn to calm himself. This issue usually arises when you're trying to get your child to sleep through the night, which is an important transition. See Chapter 1 on sleep for more discussion.

A friend of mine told me to try signing with my baby. What is this?

Initially a baby's communication tools are limited to crying and a few facial expressions. The result is often frustration and more crying. You can help reduce frustration by teaching your baby a few simple signs before he is able to verbalize the words. Most babies learn one or two signs like shaking their head or turning away to indicate *no*. They use body language naturally and smile when they're happy. Signing helps language development by teaching babies as young as nine months old additional simple gestures—such as signing *more*—to help them communicate before they are able to talk.

A longitudinal National Institutes of Health (NIH) study found that babies who learned signing beginning at eleven months were three months ahead of peers in language development by two years old, and eleven months ahead at three years old.

Parent courses in baby signing are available in many parts of the country and have even been offered by the military for servicemen's families. You can also buy books that show you how to use signing with your baby. (See the Resources section in the back of the book.) Signing is particularly helpful for late bloomers because language delay can lead to behavior problems. This system of nonverbal communication can help head off trouble as the child grows.

How can I prevent my baby from transitioning from crying to whining?

Approaching the end of the first year, babies start having opinions about things but don't have the words (or enough words) to express them. Frustration can lead to whining by the end of the second year. It's important to reduce use of crying and whining as a mode of communication by respecting the baby's body language, allowing him to use body language, and teaching simple signing. Talk to your baby, smile, make eye contact, and read to him. This is how you teach him to use and understand words.

COPING WITH COLIC

I've heard that colic causes nonstop crying that makes everyone's life miserable. What is colic?

If a baby cries uncontrollably for no apparent reason for more than three hours a day, and more than three times a week—and this continues for over three weeks—the problem could be infantile colic. Colic involves acute intestinal distress and affects about 20 percent of infants. It usually appears from out of the blue at around three weeks of age. The evening hours of 6:00 to 10:00 p.m. are often a regular crying time for infants who don't have colic, whereas babies with colic can cry for hours on end at any time of the day or night.

Colicky babies may cry right through feedings and often will refuse to feed. They'll arch their back in pain, and seem inconsolable. Clenched fists and legs drawn up are also typical. Although walking around and singing to the child ordinarily calms crying babies, this may not work if the problem is colic.

What causes colic?

The truth is, we don't really know, although there are a number of theories. One theory is that colic is caused by an immature intestinal tract that takes extra time to function smoothly. In some cases, colic symptoms are associated with an allergy to cow's milk protein in the mother's diet or in infant formula that can cause gastric distress. Reflux, which occurs when liquid from the stomach backs up into the esophagus, is believed to be another possible cause.

Because the signs of colic are nonspecific, and there can be other reasons why some babies cry so much and are inconsolable, the colic diagnosis should be made by a pedia-trician. For example, something as bizarre as a hair wrapped around the baby's toe or a small splinter can cause terrible pain. Occasionally extreme irritability can be due to neu-rologic impairment. In the end, colic is a mystery in many ways. A diagnosis can become a case of "We've ruled every-thing else out so it must be colic." Conversely, if the crying is accompanied by fever, diarrhea, or vomiting, it probably isn't colic.

When will the colic go away?

Colic usually goes away by three months of age, which would be explained by the immature intestinal tract theory. If colic symptoms continue past three months or so, there is probably another problem that must be addressed.

Are certain babies more susceptible to colic than others?

Colic is gender neutral and seems to occur in both formula-fed and breastfed babies. It appears in families seemingly randomly, although there could be a genetic component. Once we identify the exact cause of colic, we'll be better able to identify triggers.

What can be done for colic?

There is no sure cure. If a breastfed baby seems colicky, the mother may be put on a dairy-free (and possibly soy-free) diet in case the baby is allergic to cow's milk protein. Babies with a cow's milk protein allergy are often allergic to soy, too. It's worth a try even though most colicky babies don't have the allergy. A study in the journal *Pediatrics* found a significant reduction in crying time when breastfeeding moms eliminated all dairy, soy, wheat, eggs, peanuts, tree nuts, and fish from their diets. If a colicky baby is bottle

Colic Remedies around the World

Virtually every culture has used home folk remedies over the years to treat colic. Some work sometimes; some don't, but are harmless. Others can be downright dangerous. Here are some folk remedies for colic:

- Gripe water contains varying combinations of herbs such as fennel, ginger, and peppermint. This centuries-old remedy has been used in Europe (where some versions contain alcohol) and in many Asian countries, including India. There is no evidence it works, and one brand was recalled in the United States.
- Chamomile or mint tea is used in many cultures.
- Fennel water is used for colic in Asia.
- Mylicon drops (simethicone) are sometimes used in the United States. Some parents swear by the drops, although studies show they aren't any more effective than placebos.
- Catnip and the herb asafetida are used for colic in Appalachia. Catnip tea and senna abstract (castoria) may be used in the African-American culture. It may seem harmless to try a folk, herbal, or other alternative remedy when colic has made everyone's life miserable, but always check with your doctor first. Also tell caregivers these remedies are off limits unless physician-approved. Although many products *are* harmless, some are poisonous and can cause other serious health problems. For example, Greta and Azarcon are two Hispanic folk remedies for colic. They may contain as much as 90 percent lead, according to the Virginia Department of Health. Teas made from star anise are popular in many countries to help colic, but can be toxic. Outbreaks of serious

illness have been associated with star anise and there are no known scientific benefits.

Herbal and folk remedies are not regulated and ingredient concentrations can vary. Most of these remedies are imported into the United States from other countries.

fed, he is switched from regular formula to an elemental formula, which breaks down the nutrients to make them easier to tolerate. These extreme measures will only help if the crying is caused by cow's milk protein allergy or some other food sensitivity in the mother's diet.

Anti-reflux medications like Prilosec and Zantac have become very popular in recent years for cases of colic thought to be related to reflux. Occasionally, colicky babies do better with these drugs, although some data suggests they're overused.

The bright light on the horizon now is probiotics, which are bacteria beneficial to our health. Research suggests a specific probiotic called lactobacillus reuteri 55730 may be helpful for colic. A 2008 study in the journal *Pediatrics* found that by the 28th day, a group of babies taking this probiotic supplement averaged 51 minutes of crying time a day versus 145 minutes in a control group taking simethicone.

Are there other measures I can take to help colic?

Because these babies like motion, it may help to rock them or take them out for a walk or a ride in the car. Colicky infants are often very sensitive to stimuli, and a dark, quiet, calm environment may help. It's probably a mistake to expose a colicky baby to a noisy party or other event. Do your best to stay as relaxed as possible yourself, although it isn't easy. In a vicious cycle, parenting a colicky baby makes you tense—but your tension increases the baby's distress. A hot water bottle on the baby's stomach may help, but be sure to check that the water temperature is merely warm, not hot. Burp the baby every time after feeding; passing gas may help relieve the baby's discomfort.

Colic is causing lots of tension in our house. What should we do?

Colic won't harm your baby, but it can drive you up the wall. A screaming baby makes both parents feel helpless and inadequate. When the screaming continues for hours at a time and for weeks and weeks, it can result in feelings of anger and resentment. This is a normal reaction in cases of severe colic, and it's crucial to stay aware of signs that you're nearing the end of your rope. If you know your baby is tired and needs to go to sleep, it is okay to put him down and let him cry it out.

Remember to respect your limits, and take them seriously. Try to get respite care from a babysitter, grandparent, or other caretaker. Colic is very hard to cope with and no parent is a saint. Support from your pediatrician, family, and/or friends can also help. If you feel out of control or depressed, however, it's time to seek professional counseling. It's sad but true that colicky babies can be at risk for child abuse.

LEARNING FROM TEARS

Crying is your baby's way of communicating with you. Learning to interpret cries and cues, and figuring out how to respond appropriately, is critical to your baby's emo-

Talking Together

Most babies are able to sleep through the night by four or five months if they're allowed to self-soothe, which initially begins with crying. There is usually one parent who can't stand the baby crying and will go in and "rescue" her. Rescuers aren't able to teach self-soothing, which is an important developmental skill for babies. Because that's the way rescuers are wired, the other spouse had better be able to set some limits to prevent dysfunctional sleep patterns from overtaking the household. One couple turned to the husband's mother to arbitrate. Says the wife: "I'm the tough one in the family, but my husband always gives in after two minutes. We fought about it, but his mother supported me, and I won out."

Sleep training is your first experience in setting limits—obviously a very gentle limit setting. Talk together about your respective strengths and challenges when the baby cries and how you can complement each other. Some people are good at limit setting; others are not, but have other parenting talents.

At the other end of the spectrum, we all have emotions and we all get overtired and stressed. Even infants can push our buttons, and you may put down a baby screaming for hours more harshly than you should. That's less likely to happen if you and your spouse discuss in advance how to handle the situation. Then you can agree, "We're not going to do that." Raise your awareness, and talk about options when you start to feel you're "losing it." You may decide you'll call a friend or relative to vent. Or maybe you'll say, "We're at our wits' end and need a break. Let's get a babysitter." A break from your baby is not selfish or a sign you're a failure as a parent.

tional and neurological development. But it takes time to become comfortable and confident about understanding baby language. Be kind to yourself and don't expect to master these skills overnight. With patience, awareness, and the ability to ask for help when you need it, you're going to do just fine.

CHAPTER 5

Pee, Poop, and Spit-Ups— The Diaper Diaries

This chapter covers:

- All about voiding and urine
- Diaper rashes and how to handle them
- Stooling, diarrhea, and constipation
- When it's time to call the doctor
- Spit-ups and vomiting

As new parents, you're probably going to spend an inordinate amount of time focusing on the details of your baby's bodily functions. It's simply that parents develop their own ideas of what constitutes normal pee and poop—and equate them with good health. Misunderstandings often follow, with needless worry and, sometimes, unnecessary interventions. Spit-ups are another issue.

Here are the common questions I hear on this topic. The answers will educate you to what is really normal and how to handle symptoms that need attention.

VOIDING

How often should my baby wet her diaper?

Most newborns void eleven to sixteen times a day, but there are variations. Please don't count unless your pediatrician is concerned about dehydration (depletion of the baby's body fluids). Diapers today are so absorbent that it may be hard to know whether the baby has actually urinated. Often urine is mixed with stool, which also makes it difficult to tell. There are two times when tracking urine output is important: the first days of breastfeeding before the mother's milk supply is

established, and when the baby is ill, especially if fever, excessive vomiting, or diarrhea causes increased fluid output.

What should I do if my baby hasn't wet for eight hours?

This can indicate dehydration, which can be a high risk situation for a newborn and even life threatening. Other signs
of dehydration include a dry mouth, listlessness, irritability,
and a depressed fontanel (soft spot on the top of the skull).
Dehydration may occur in the first two or three days after
the baby comes home. That's one reason why doctors like to
see babies within forty-eight hours of leaving the hospital.

Babies become dehydrated in two ways: either they take
in an inadequate amount of fluid or they excrete too much. If
you suspect your baby is dehydrated, call your pediatrician.

How is dehydration treated in a newborn?

First, the breastfeeding technique must be evaluated. If the
baby is not latching on properly, she may not be getting
enough milk, and she may not be stimulating the breast
properly to increase the milk supply. Possibly a lactation
consultant will be recommended. Occasionally breastfeeding is supplemented with formula, usually temporarily, to
provide more fluids. Because dehydration is a serious medical matter, your pediatrician (rather than the lactation consultant or your spouse) should be the one to help you with
this decision.

What does normal baby urine look like?

It is pale yellow and remains that color as the infant gets
older. A change in color usually reflects the concentration
of the urine. For example, the paler the yellow, the more
hydrated the baby. Very deep yellow urine is a sign the baby
is mildly dehydrated. Liver disease, urinary tract infections
(UTIs), and metabolic problems can also affect the color
and odor of the urine.

My baby's urine sometimes seems to have a strong odor. Why?

Normal baby urine should not have a strong odor. This is definitely something you should discuss with your doctor. Often the odor is due to mild dehydration where the urine is concentrated. Another possibility is a urinary tract infection. Estimated UTI incidence ranges as high as 7.5 percent in the first three months of life.

Less likely causes of strong odor are certain metabolic conditions that can cause a fruity or other unusual smell. Your baby will have received a screening for most metabolic disorders on discharge from the hospital nursery.

When I change my baby's diaper I see little crystals. What are they?

In the first few weeks of life, babies' urine can contain small crystals. These are usually uric acid and are normal. The crystals may be clear, orange, or salmon color. Another possibility is these crystals come from the diaper, not the urine. Sometimes new absorbent disposable diapers contain a hygroscopic gel, such as silica gel, that can crystallize. Ignore it.

I saw blood and mucus on my newborn's diaper when I changed her. What could this be?

Right after birth, female babies sometimes experience a little menstrual period due to hormones they have received from the mother. The "period" doesn't last long and usually involves a very small amount of blood. Tell the doctor if blood in the urine occurs after the first week of life.

How long is too long for my baby to be left in a wet diaper?

Ideally, you should change a diaper as soon as you know it's wet. The longer it's on the baby, the likelier it is that a rash will develop.

What You Should Know about Diaper Rashes

Most diaper rashes are a form of diaper dermatitis that can be caused by infrequent diaper changes. Basically, wet urine on skin may cause an inflammatory reaction. Certain foods such as tomatoes can also cause a response. Other diaper rashes can be due to yeast or bacteria, and even, sometimes, chemicals in the wipes you use to clean the diaper area.

Diaper rashes can vary in appearance:

Diaper dermatitis from infrequent changes looks red and may form little red bumps. Rashes from certain foods look red, almost like a burn, and appear right after a stool. The best treatment is prevention, but if it's too late for that, thick emollients with lanolin and zinc oxide—the ingredients in most over-the-counter diaper creams—work. Occasionally a steroid cream may be added by your doctor.

Bacterial rashes may have pustules. There may be areas that are peeling. Treatment is either a topical antibiotic or perhaps an oral antibiotic from your doctor.

Yeast rash is usually red and raised with little satellite lesions. Yeast loves a warm moist environment, and diapers are the perfect greenhouse. This rash is particularly likely to occur after the baby receives a course of antibiotics for something else. Why? Because yeast normally occurs on the skin but is kept in check by skin bacteria. Antibiotics may eliminate some of these "good" bacteria, allowing the yeast to multiply and cause a rash. This is a fungal rash. Your doctor will write a prescription for an anti-fungal cream to treat it. Sometimes the baby has yeast in his mouth or intestinal tract. Every time he poops, the diaper area is reseeded with yeast. In this case, you may need both a topical anti-fungal cream and an oral anti-fungal medication.

Many parents feel guilty when they show me a rash because they think it reflects negatively on their parenting. Not to worry. All babies get a rash occasionally, and fair babies are prone to them. It has nothing to do with you as long as you clean and change the baby regularly.

Do I need to wake up the baby at night to change a diaper?

"Never wake a sleeping baby" is a mantra I repeat, even at the risk of diaper rash. Diapers today are quite absorbent, and you don't have to change a wet one in the middle of the night. If the baby has pooped, that's different. She will probably wake up and let you know. If she doesn't, and you can smell the poop, you should still change it, even if that means waking the baby up. After an hour or so, a poopy diaper will cause a rash. Be especially diligent if your baby has very fair skin that is susceptible to rashes. In that case, it's important to get both wet and poopy diapers off the skin. Diaper creams containing lanolin and zinc oxide can help put a barrier between the baby's skin and excretions.

STOOLING

When do babies have their first poop?

This usually takes place during or right after birth. The first stool, which is called meconium, is sticky and black. Meconium is usually followed by yellow seedy stool for several weeks, especially in breastfed babies.

How often should my baby poop?

The frequency of bowel movements can vary. Some babies poop every time they feed. Food reaching the stomach triggers the gastro-colic reflex, which causes the colon to contract and produce a bowel movement. Because newborns have a very sensitive gastro-colic reflex, they poop after feeding more than older babies do. Other babies may not have a movement for forty-eight to seventy-two hours on occasion.

What constitutes diarrhea in a newborn?

Diarrhea is abnormal frequency or liquidity of fecal discharge. It's very hard to diagnose diarrhea in a newborn without looking at other body functions. For example, because newborns normally have frequent watery stools, you have to look for other signs, such as vomiting, loss of appetite, and maybe cramping, fussiness, or listlessness. A viral or bacterial infection can cause diarrhea, but other stressors can lead to loose stools in babies, as well.

Why does my baby have green stools?

Green stool contains bile, which the liver secretes into the small intestine. If the bile is not absorbed by the intestine, it is excreted in stool. Green stool reflects transit time (the speed at which stool is excreted). Sometimes fast transit time doesn't give bile a chance to be absorbed. This is nothing to worry about.

Certain solid foods, such as beets (red) and peas (green), or foods with food coloring can also change the color of stool.

My baby has blood in her stool. Why does this happen?

If blood appears in stool, the most common cause is cow's milk protein allergy. See Chapter 12 for information on this allergy. Your doctor may discontinue all dairy products (and possibly soy) in the breastfeeding mother's diet to see if bleeding stops. Formula-fed babies may be changed to an elemental formula, where the protein has been broken down and is more easily digestible. If bleeding continues, your doctor may refer you to a gastroenterologist.

Sometimes stool can look bright red, due to bleeding from a small fissure or crack near the rectum, caused by severe diaper rash or hard stool. The doctor may prescribe a stool softener or tell you to put the baby on diluted prune juice to allow the fissure to heal.

Are there other stool colors I should know about?

Alert your doctor to black stool that appears anytime other than in the newborn period. Black tarry stool may reflect bleeding high up in the intestines. White stool, which is rare, may reflect a liver problem.

My baby's poop looks different from that of my neighbor's baby. Is it because my baby is breastfed and hers isn't?

Yes. Formula-fed babies can have slightly more formed stools and they may poop less frequently than breastfed babies. Keep in mind both are considered normal.

Is it true breastfed babies are less likely to be constipated than bottle-fed babies?

Generally yes, but part of the equation is the genetics of gut motility. Sometimes there's a genetic tendency to have very slow motility. If you or your spouse has a sluggish gut, your baby may stool less.

What is considered constipation in a baby?

Constipation—which is difficult or infrequent evacuation of feces—may occur in babies, whether they're breast- or formula-fed. Babies are not considered constipated unless there's blood in the stool, the stool is hard, and/or the baby cries in pain when pooping.

My baby often turns red and strains a lot when he has a bowel movement. Is that okay?

It's normal for babies to be red in the face and strain to stool. Pooping while lying on one's back requires increased intra-abdominal pressure and a certain amount of exertion.

Why does my baby cry when she has a bowel movement?

Crying is not normal when stooling and must be checked out by your pediatrician. We never want babies to experience pain while pooping or they'll associate evacuation with discomfort and try to hold back bowel movements when they get older. This issue becomes more important in the second year after toilet training begins. Crying may indicate gas is pushing along in the colon when she strains, or she has a little tear in the rectum, which is possible if the baby is constipated and is straining a lot.

What can I do to help my constipated baby?

Check with your pediatrician first because there are many different ways to handle constipation in babies. Your child may need more fluid, and your doctor will weigh the baby to check on this and ask about urination frequency. Or the doctor may prescribe a stool softener. My personal preference after age two months is to dilute two ounces of prune juice with an equal amount of sterilized tap water. You can also buy diluted baby prune juice. If your baby is on solid food, switch him from rice cereal (which is binding) to oatmeal or barley cereal, and avoid bananas and applesauce. Instead, substitute pureed apricots or prunes. If the baby is eating table food, cantaloupe and raisins are good fruits. Avoid cheese, rice, and pastas.

Family members may recommend folk remedies for constipation, but always run the idea past your pediatrician before trying one. Such remedies are not regulated. For example, ghasard, an ayurvedic medicine given to constipated babies in India and in areas of the United States with certain Asian immigrant populations, contains lead.

What's the best kind of diaper to use?

Diapers that wrap around legs snugly enough to prevent any leakage, but not too tightly to be tolerated, are the best. Beyond that, there are pros and cons to disposable and cloth diapers. Disposables are costly but convenient. New versions of cloth diapers use Velcro closures instead of pins and have water repellent covers that replace rubber pants, which often caused diaper rash. But laundry is an issue. Environmentally friendly or "green" diapers are also available.

How gentle must we be when cleaning the baby's bottom?

Usually, the nurse at the hospital goes over basic diaper hygiene with you. Parents sometimes overdo the cleaning, and that is more of a problem than not cleaning enough, especially for girls. Treat the vaginal area gently when cleaning off stool in a girl. The vaginal area is fragile because baby girls do not have enough estrogen to protect it. Wipe the rectal area and clean stool from the vaginal area without being overly aggressive. You can always wash off stool from that area with water or a bath, if necessary. Avoid using baby powder, as babies can inhale it. If your baby is prone to rashes, use diaper cream.

My coworker is from China and is toilet training her one year old baby. Is it possible to do that so young?

In many parts of Asia, as well as some African, Latin American, and other countries, toilet training for babies begins very early, sometimes as early as the first weeks of life. In some cultures babies are trained by a year old. In the United States and Western Europe, the starting time tends to be around eighteen months, although many families start later. I believe there's no reason in our culture to tackle toilet training before the child is ready. You'll know he is ready when he expresses interest or lets you know when he starts to pee or poop. It takes a lot of time and trouble to train early. It's so much easier to wait. Fortunately, today most day care centers have relaxed their requirements for timing of toilet training.

Red Flag Signs That Say, "Call the Doctor"

- Blood in stool
- White stool
- Black stool
- Hard stools that make the baby cry
- Blood in urine
- Foul odor to urine
- No urination for more than eight hours
- Repeated voluminous vomiting
- Green vomit
- Spitting up and turning blue
- Spitting up every feeding

SPIT-UP

Why do babies spit up?

All babies spit up some milk during the first three months of life. This regurgitation is also known as gastroesophageal reflux (known as GER), which is the backward flow of stomach contents into the esophagus. As food travels down the esophagus and enters the stomach, a muscle or sphincter prevents food from backing up. In the first three months, the muscle is still immature and not yet working properly. Food is easily regurgitated. That muscle naturally tightens up over time. By the end of the first year, most babies have stopped spitting up.

My baby never used to spit up. Now he does it all the time. Why?

You may not see a lot of spitting up in a newborn because the baby is often taking a small volume of nourishment and is not moving around much. Increased milk intake and greater mobility as he grows cause more regurgitation or GER.

Why do I sometimes see milk coming out of my baby's nose?

Occasionally regurgitation is forceful enough to propel the milk out of both the mouth and nose. This is normal. If the milk is not sneezed out, you can clear the nose with a bulb syringe bought at the drug store.

Are there ways to prevent spitting up?

Overfeeding your baby can cause spit-ups, which is one reason why pushing the baby to finish a bottle is a bad idea. You can also hold the bottle at a slant to facilitate constant flow and discourage air intake. Over the years people have tried a number of other techniques. One of them is to keep the baby upright and immobile for twenty to sixty minutes in a car seat or infant chair after feeding. Another is to thicken formula with baby cereal after four months of age. I've found that neither of these is very effective, but with the permission of your pediatrician you can try them if you wish.

Burping during and after feeding may help. Parents often think they must get a burp out after every feeding to prevent gas. My advice is to burp the baby for a few seconds. If the burp doesn't come up quickly, try changing positions—

to your shoulder or face down on your lap—to bring the air bubble out. But don't spend a lot of time on it. The burp is either there or it's not. If the bubble is too far down to come out now, it will come out later. You can also slightly elevate the head of the crib mattress (if the baby isn't rolling yet) to keep his head higher than his feet.

My friend's doctor gave her baby medicine for spitting up. Should I get some to keep on hand?

This is a discussion to have with your pediatrician. Currently some pediatricians use acid blockers such as Zantac to treat GER when the baby tends to be very fussy. The thinking is that heartburn, which is painful, is accompanying reflux. In my experience, acid blockers have rarely been helpful in this particular situation. There's a general consensus that they're overused for something physiologic that will go away by itself.

Should we change my baby to a lactose-free formula because she is spitting up too much on regular formula?

There's really no reason to change formula because she's spitting up. If there's concern that spit-ups are caused by cow's milk protein allergy, usually there are signs of blood and mucus in the stool, as well. This condition should be diagnosed by your pediatrician, an allergist, or gastroenterologist, who might put the baby on an appropriate elemental formula such as Neutramogen, Neocate, or Progestamil. A lactose-free formula won't help because the problem is not lactose intolerance. Random formula changes are not helpful and may cause diarrhea or constipation, which will present another problem to deal with.

What's the difference between vomiting and spitting up?

It can sometimes be hard to tell the difference. The amount that comes up is one clue. Vomiting is usually more forceful and may produce old undigested food. Spitting up is generally not very forceful, and results in offering up a recent feeding. On the other hand, sometimes an air bubble in the stomach behind food can result in spit-up that is quite profuse and projectile.

Even reflux can produce old curdled milk that has not yet been fully digested.

What causes vomiting?

Vomiting may be a sign of illness and needs to be addressed. A stomach virus is possible, especially if other household members are ill. In such cases, other symptoms may be present, such as fever, diarrhea, fussiness, lethargy, loss of appetite. Or, the trouble may be that food disagrees with the baby. And sometimes vomiting signals an allergy to cow's milk protein. Babies may also vomit due to constipation or simple overheating in the summer.

A condition called pyloric stenosis can also cause vomiting. Some babies around the age of six weeks, for reasons that are unclear, develop a thickening of the sphincter muscle at the end of the stomach near the small intestine. The thickening can form a blockage that must be opened up via surgery. These babies are sick, vomit all feedings all the time, and look ill. There may be green bile in the vomit. Pyloric stenosis is more common in boys than girls. Other causes of obstruction include congenital abnormalities. These usually turn up in the first weeks of life.

Repeated vomiting can lead to dehydration, and may indicate trauma, infection, increased pressure in the brain, or a metabolic problem.

Can spitting up be dangerous?

If the baby is gaining weight and growing and there's no blood in her stool and no recurrent pneumonias, then reflux is part of normal physiology. Spitting up is usually not dangerous in a neurologically intact baby. Any danger would involve choking on or aspirating the spit-up. If stomach contents come up and enter the trachea or breathing tube, the baby could choke. In neurologically healthy babies, this rarely happens—and if it does, the baby's cough or gag reflex should clear the spit-up from the airway. To aid that response, sit him up. If you have a healthy baby who spits up a lot, talk to your pediatrician, who will want to check on weight gain, signs of respiratory distress, or blood in the stool.

Babies with certain neurologic conditions such as cerebral palsy may have a gag response that is not intact. They can choke and aspirate, and they get recurrent pneumonia as food travels into the lungs.

My baby is vomiting green. What should I do?

This is called bilious vomiting and may indicate a blockage somewhere. This type of vomiting should always be reported to your doctor.

What about blood in the vomit?

In the first days after birth, babies may spit up blood. This is usually blood the baby has swallowed during passage through the birth canal. After the first days of life, blood in the vomit of a breastfed baby could be blood from the mother's cracked nipple. Blood in vomit may also signal bleeding in the gastrointestinal tract and is potentially serious. Always tell your doctor about it.

Why do babies get gas?

Gas is air that's swallowed when babies cry, eat, and just live. The air will bubble up with burping or may come up on its own. If it passes along the intestine, it may be absorbed along the way or be passed as rectal gas. Gas can be caused by normal bacteria that are part of intestinal flora as they break down food products such as milk. Some babies have more gas than others.

Babies cry because they have gas at times, but it becomes a chicken and egg problem. As they cry they swallow more air, which causes more gas. It can be confusing.

Talking Together

Parents tend to obsess over the baby's body functions, and it's helpful to look at the answers in this chapter together. A review will clarify what is normal and what is not and will help avoid disagreements about whether the baby is constipated or spitting up way too much. Discussion will also reveal whether your upbringing is playing a role in how you perceive your child's health. Some parents feel overanxious and make a record of every poop long after the early weeks. Others are more laid back.

Talk together about diaper duty, as well. Most couples I see today come up with a plan to divide some of the less pleasant tasks. Many use a team approach and take turns changing dirty diapers. But some couples report that dad opts out. Why? This baby belongs to both of you.

You may also want to discuss how both of you feel about toilet training. Some cultures believe the baby should be trained by a year old, and there may pressure from relatives to do so. I try to get couples to relax about this issue, and often quote the adage, "Nobody goes to college in diapers."

LIFE IS MESSY

Daily interactions with the contents of diapers and/or the remnants of partially digested meals are among the many changes in your household since your baby arrived. Stooling, voiding, and spit-ups have become important markers for parents worried about their baby's health. Fortunately, most of the time your pediatrician can provide perspective and relieve anxieties about what is normal and what is not.

CHAPTER 6

Growth and Development— A Wide Range of Normal

This chapter covers:

- Vital statistics: weight, height, and evaluating growth
- Motor development
- Milestones
- Autism
- Stimulation to enhance development
- Tests for newborns
- Well-baby visits

An amazing amount of growth and change occurs during the first year of your baby's life, and it's only human to worry whether your child is on track. It's hard to tune out the cacophony of warnings to detect developmental delay early—warnings that are fueled by the increase in autism in recent years. Yet I can assure you that what's normal covers a lot of territory. Genes, personality, and differences in physical activity, concentration, and motivation can all make an impact on whether your baby reaches certain milestones early, late, or right on time. In most cases, parents' anxieties about the pace of progress and what it portends are groundless.

Following are the most frequent questions new parents ask me about growth and development. The answers will help you understand how pediatricians evaluate babies, and what is or isn't cause for concern.

WEIGHT, HEIGHT, AND OTHER MEASUREMENTS

How do I know whether my baby is growing normally?

Your pediatrician or family physician will measure three parameters for your baby's growth: height, weight, and head circumference. Growth in each of these three areas will be recorded and checked with growth charts based on national standards for age and gender. These charts are updated periodically to adjust for changing demographics in the United States.

We look for reassurance that the baby continues to grow, and we track progress from birth, from the last visit, and from the one before that.

How much weight should my baby gain?

Babies normally lose weight in the nursery before coming home from the hospital. This loss, which should not exceed 10 percent of body weight, is regained after about ten days. Babies tend to gain about one to two pounds a month in the first six months, and a pound per month in the second six months. Try not to be rigid about these numbers because they're intended merely as guidelines. Genetics, cultural differences, and feeding methods can and do cause variations.

What if my baby doesn't gain weight or grow taller?

Lack of weight gain alerts the doctor there's a problem. Babies who don't gain weight either aren't taking in enough calories or have increased output due to diarrhea or a metabolic problem, or they may have trouble absorbing nutrients. An overactive thyroid could be responsible, or the baby may have a fever and be ill. A viral illness can also cause babies to lose weight, although they quickly gain the weight back.

Failure to grow properly in height could be due to a hormone deficiency, a genetic defect, insufficient calorie intake, or a metabolic problem. In general, babies should grow about an inch a month in the first six months, and half an inch a month in the next six months. But remember those genes. These are just rough guidelines.

What does my baby's "percentile" mean?

Percentiles are a device pediatricians use to evaluate babies' growth relative to peers of the same age and gender. For example, a two-and-a-half-month-old girl may be in the 75th percentile for length. That means she is taller than 75 percent of females the same age. If a six-and-a-half-month-old boy is in the 25th percentile for weight, he weighs more than 25 percent of male babies his age.

The goal is to keep the percentiles for weight and length balanced. A baby in the 50th percentile for weight and the 25th percentile for height could be too chubby unless he is muscular. In the first year of life it is difficult to overfeed your baby, especially if you are following guidelines from your doctor for food selection and volume. Many times I ask parents to find old baby pictures of themselves and compare their body type at that age with their baby's. Usually the body types are similar. Percentiles may spotlight a worrisome trend, but let your doctor interpret the numbers for you before you put your baby on a treadmill. A diagnosis of "failure to thrive" suggests that the child has fallen below the 5th percentile for weight for a period of time.

Keep in mind that your child's percentile is merely an assessment tool. If you and your spouse are short, there's a good chance your baby will be short, too. The gene pool is the determinant. At every well-baby visit, I give parents a sheet listing the child's weight, length, head circumference, and percentile for that visit and for previous visits. This sheet shows the baby's progress in concrete terms. If the doctor doesn't provide such information automatically, ask for it and write it down.

Why is head circumference important?

Doctors measure babies' heads up to about twelve to fifteen months of age, and check a percentile chart as part of the assessment. We want to know whether the head is growing too rapidly, too slowly, or not at all. Rapid growth can indicate increased pressure inside the skull from a tumor, a congenital defect, or an endocrine problem, but it is commonly a genetic issue. Big heads may run in the family. A head that is not growing at all is a sign of microcephaly (or "small head"), which suggests a genetic disorder or fetal alcohol syndrome.

Does our family's cultural background affect growth norms?

Yes, and we take them into consideration. Normal height for an Asian baby might be less than for a child of Scandinavian parents. On the other hand, there are tall Asian babies. If the family tends to be tall, the baby is usually tall. But there could be one aunt who's tiny. Genetic expression is complex. There are no growth charts based on ethnicity, but the charts we use are based on nationwide statistics that reflect the new immigrant pools.

Are premature babies assessed with the same charts?

Yes, but we subtract the number of months of prematurity. For example, a baby born two months ago who was one month premature is assessed as a one-month-old on growth charts.

How long will the doctor continue to use growth charts for my child?

Growth charts will probably still be used until the end of puberty, which occurs around age seventeen or eighteen for boys, and sixteen or seventeen for girls, but could be slightly earlier or later. Adolescents are considered fully grown at this time.

How can I prevent my baby from getting fat?

If your child looks chubby before solid food is added to his diet (usually by four or five months), it's probably just a phase. Ask your doctor whether you're overfeeding. Perhaps you're mistaking cries for attention for hunger. But it's more likely that this is his body type, predetermined by genes.

The situation changes once solid foods begin, and it's important to respect your baby's signals. If she turns her head away, signaling that she's finished, accept that rather than push a jar or a dish at her to encourage her to finish. Most babies know when they've had enough, although every so often I encounter one who seems to lack a satiety center. In that case, your doctor will give you rough guidelines on how much to feed her.

Be aware, too, that babies take less breast milk or formula after solids are added to the diet. Expect reduced milk intake. In fact, doctors worry if a child takes more than thirty-two ounces at this transition. Your pediatrician will watch very carefully for signs of excessive weight gain after solids begin.

Keep in mind that it may be tempting to overfeed a baby who cries a great deal, as a quieting device. Try not to make a habit of offering unnecessary calories in this way. Similarly, do not restrict calories for your baby if you are obsessed about weight.

Why is my baby chubby even though she eats normally?

Some babies do not overeat, yet are naturally pudgy. Were you pudgy yourself at that age? As chubby babies become more mobile and grow taller, they usually thin out. Some babies are naturally very active and burn calories by moving a lot. Others are relaxed, mellow, and relatively stationary. If put down in one spot, they stay there. This does not mean they're doomed to be fat adults.

Do doctors consider BMI when evaluating weight?

As your baby gets older, the doctor may add another percentile to follow—the body mass index (BMI). BMI is thought to be more reliable than height and weight as a measurement of excess body fat. Doctors don't use BMI until a child passes two years of age. Technically, a child is overweight if the BMI is 25 to 30 and obese if over 30.

Is there anything I can do to make my baby grow taller?

No, not aside from good nutrition. Years ago, growth hormone was in vogue to help short children grow. Today, growth hormone treatment is not considered medically sound unless there is a medical reason for it, such as a hormone deficiency. Growth hormone is also very expensive.

MOTOR DEVELOPMENT

When should my baby be able to hold his head up?

Even some newborns will lift their heads a bit when placed face down on the mother's chest, but most will start by one month and begin to look around. Take care to support the neck and head when picking up your baby.

When can I stop supporting my baby's head?

When you see that she can keep her head up by herself, which usually occurs around three or four months of age, you can stop supporting her head and neck when picking her up. It does depend on the child.

When is it safe to start using a stroller?

Not until five or six months of age when babies start sitting up unsupported. It isn't until about six to nine months that most babies really sit without support. You can use a stroller earlier if you want, but then you must prop the baby up to prevent flopping over.

Why does the doctor say my baby needs "tummy time"?

Because babies now sleep on their back, they don't get much upper body or arm exercise. As a result, those muscles are pretty weak. Hand, wrist, arm, and shoulder muscles need exercise too. Start tummy time once your baby is old enough to be on his stomach during playtime. This is usually after four weeks of age, when infants can push on their arms. Begin with several minutes on the tummy, and gradually increase the time as tolerated. Some babies start screaming right away. They get frustrated because they can't see what's going on. Eventually they get used to it, especially if there are objects or a human face to entertain them in this position. If your infant still screams after five or ten minutes, switch him over to his back again. This is a time to use your judgment. Tummy time also helps prevent infants from developing a flat head due to sleeping on their backs in one spot. See Chapter 1 for more information.

When should my baby start to roll over?

We used to expect babies to roll over by four months of age, but that was when infants slept on their stomachs. Now we know sleeping on the back can help prevent SIDS, and today most babies sleep in that position. Because it's harder to turn from the back position to the stomach than it is to roll from the stomach to the back, many babies roll over later than they used to. I now give a four- to six-month window of time to reach this milestone. Tummy time helps to strengthen the upper body and allows babies to roll both ways.

Larger babies (who have a bigger body mass to move) often are slower to roll over than smaller infants.

> ### Babies' Personalities
>
> Be who you are, but recognize that your child may be different. I've found that babies have their own personalities from day one. Some are quiet and manageable; others cry a great deal. Some are active and energetic; others are laid back. Mellow babies love to be naked. Very sensitive or colicky babies hate it. But I believe environment counts as well. A family that travels out and about encourages openness to new experiences. A household suspicious of strangers sends a different message. Children pick up on these things.

The doctor mentioned my baby has good tone. What does "tone" mean?

Tone refers to a general sense of how the baby holds himself. A newborn is like a floppy blob of jelly. But some newborns have amazing head control if you lift them. Some are very quick to roll over. Babies can be "hypotonic" or "hypertonic." Hypotonic babies tend to be slow to perform their motor milestones. Often they are content, low maintenance babies who are not particularly motivated to roll over, crawl, or walk. In contrast, hypertonic babies are muscular, active babies who seem to hit their motor milestones quickly—sometimes even early. Both types of babies are usually normal, but a doctor who thinks your baby is sluggish or slow may check for low thyroid, genetic anomalies, or a developmental problem. If your baby is very jittery and hypertonic, he may be checked for cerebral palsy or a metabolic problem. In between is a huge range of normal.

When should my baby start crawling?

Babies can start moving around as early as four months. But they don't actually crawl until anywhere from six to ten months. Motivation is a factor in when they begin. Some babies are very content and don't care if they can get to a toy or not. They're happy to play with whatever is around. On the other hand, some hyperactive babies just have to get to objects right away.

My baby inches along on his belly instead of crawling on hands and knees like other babies I see. Why?

This is called a commando crawl and is one of several variations of crawling that babies can adopt. These variations are normal and nothing to worry about. Most babies crawl before they stand, but there are also some "vertically inclined babies," who skip crawling altogether and just stand up one day.

When should my baby start walking?

Babies may start walking anywhere from eight-and-a-half to twelve months, although some can walk with assistance as early as six months. Some babies are very cautious and don't want to let go of a piece of furniture; others are adventurous. Of course a baby who walks late might do so due to an orthopedic or developmental problem. If your child is very late, your doctor will be checking to make sure a medical issue isn't hindering mobility.

In her book, *The Developing Person through Childhood and Adolescence,* Kathleen Stassen Berger, textbook author and chair and professor of the social sciences department at Bronx Community College (City University of New York), notes that Uganda seems to have the earliest walkers on the globe; healthy babies typically walk at ten months. On the other hand, French babies tend to take their first steps alone at fifteen months, and are the latest walkers.

Developmental Milestones in the First Year

Developmental milestones are skills babies develop in the course of normal growth. Here are some major ones:

Newborn

At birth we look at reflexes, which are involuntary physical responses to stimulus. The presence of certain reflexes at birth signals normal brain and neurological development, such as:

- Moro reflex, or "startle response" (a noise causes the baby to fling out arms and legs, and then flex them inward)
- Placing or walking reflex (baby takes a step when feet touch the ground)
- Stepping reflex (baby's foot lifts when a hand is placed on top of foot)
- Rooting reflex (baby turns head to suck when cheek is stroked)
- Baby lifts head slightly when placed on parent's chest
- Baby grasps object when placed in his hand

As the baby grows, I assess gross motor skills involving the large muscles of the arms, legs, etc., and fine motor skills that use the fingers and hands, as well as language, social, and cognitive skills (interacting, understanding, etc.). There are many nuances in each of these areas. Some milestones include:

One Month

- May smile
- May coo
- Lifts head up and turns it side to side when placed on stomach

Two Months
- Smiles
- Laughs
- Coos
- Studies mobile or close objects

Four Months
- May roll over
- Reaches for objects
- Puts objects and hands in mouth
- Vocalizes (makes sounds)
- Almost no head lag when pulled to sitting position

Six Months
- Sits with support
- Rolls back-to-stomach and stomach-to-back
- Brings hands together
- Transfers objects from one hand to another
- May babble (gibberish)
- Stranger anxiety and separation anxiety may begin
- May bear weight when placed in standing position

Nine Months
- Sits alone
- May crawl or creep
- Good pincer grasp
- May pull to stand
- Babbles
- May play "peek-a-boo"

Twelve Months
- May walk
- May pull to stand

- May cruise (hold onto furniture and walk)
- Recognizes own name
- May say a few words
- Waves "bye bye"
- Claps
- May respond to simple commands like "Where's Daddy?"

There are many other milestones, as well. For a more detailed look at first year milestones, check www.cdc .gov/ncbddd/actearly/interactive/milestones Remember there is a wide range of normal in milestones. It's important not to focus on any one developmental issue. Differences don't have any long-term implications unless a child is really impaired.

When will I know what hand my baby prefers?

Babies rarely show hand preference before six to nine months of age, and preference can vacillate later. Most babies will often hold something with one hand and manipulate it with the other. However, babies do tend to prefer turning to the right; if they turn to the left they may be left-handed. A clear preference doesn't emerge until age three or four years in many children.

At what age should my infant be able to grasp or pick up a toy?

This involves fine motor skills (as opposed to large motor skills involved in locomotion). Babies can start grasping in the first month. Even a newborn can grip an object if it is placed in her hand, but at this stage it is a reflex. Babies begin to hold or grasp objects with their whole hand at around four to six months. At about nine months, they develop a pincer grasp, which allows them to pick up a small object like a Cheerio with two fingers

AUTISM

How can you tell if a baby is autistic?

Autism spectrum disorder is a description of a wide range of behaviors that vary from mild language delay and social withdrawal to severe cognitive and behavioral disorders. Some children exhibit odd repetitive behaviors. Diagnosing autism is complex and can take time, as children develop along varying timelines. There's some evidence autism can be recognized at five or six months of age, but it's very unusual to find it that soon. Usually the earliest detection is in the second year.

Although the goal for doctors and parents is early diagnosis, the variability of autism's presentation and the tremendous variations in childhood development makes this goal challenging. There are new tools such as the M-CHAT (Modified Checklist for Autism in Toddlers) test, which includes questions such as "Does your baby make eye contact with you?" This test, which is used at sixteen to thirty months, will help doctors pick up autism earlier. But the most important tool is close observation and communication between doctor and families.

What causes autism?

I wish we knew. Most likely, the disorder is inherited, and scientists are focusing on genetic links that may give us an answer. There has been concern that the MMR (measles, mumps, rubella) vaccine or thimerosol, a mercury preservative once used in vaccines, contributed to the rise in autism. Many studies, however, have shown no link between the two. See Chapter 9 for further discussion of autism.

Stimulation That Enhances Your Baby's Development

Although your baby's development is governed to a large degree by genes, temperament, and other factors beyond your control, there's a great deal you can do to encourage motor and cognitive skills, such as:

- Smile at and talk to your baby. Look him in the eye as much as possible, beginning at birth.
- Address him by name. It's personal face-to-face interaction that encourages development, not videos.
- Read, read, read. From two months on, you can read simple nursery rhymes that accustom your baby to tone and language. As early as three months you can use books with sensory stimuli (for instance *Pat the Bunny)* that allow her to touch textures, see bright colors, or hear "moo." Reading also encourages intimate time with your baby.
- Play music (any kind, as long as it's soothing) and sing to the baby. Singing often can calm a crying baby, no matter how bad your voice is.
- Dance with the baby, especially if he's bored. Babies are natural dancers.
- Give plenty of floor time to provide opportunities to explore and master skills. Babies need opportunities for milestones to occur. Infants who are constantly carried around or sitting in the car or in strollers all day may not have enough chances. This is another reason baby walkers aren't recommended. They're not only dangerous; in my opinion they also impede independence and ambulation. See Chapter 11 for information on baby walkers.
- Change the environment and take the baby outside often

And don't forget to have fun. Laughing and playing together helps stimulate cognitive and social development.

My baby doesn't seem to make eye contact with me. Is this a sign of autism?

Bombarded by all the attention to autism today, many parents worry that their baby has a symptom of the condition, such as lack of eye contact. However, some healthy babies seem to dislike intense one-on-one engagement and avert their eyes. In itself, this is not a worrisome sign unless it persists, although it's something your doctor will monitor. If the baby continues avoiding eye contact or any social connection, there may be concern.

If you find yourself worrying about a developmental milestone, report your concern to the doctor. Remember, nobody spends as much time with your baby as you do; the doctor only sees her for a short time. If concerns continue, the baby will usually be sent to a developmental pediatrician or a pediatric neurologist for further evaluation.

My baby is one month old and doesn't have a social smile. Why?

Are you smiling at (and interacting with) your baby? I think babies often mimic the environment they're in. It's also possible that you just have a very serious baby, just as there are sober adults. In any case, try to avoid looking at month-to-month milestones as absolutes. Some babies don't start smiling until the end of the second month.

LANGUAGE, HEARING, VISION

When should my baby start talking?

Some babies say a word or two at nine months; others can be closer to fifteen months before they start talking, although they should be babbling with "mama" and "dada" sounds by about a year. Some babies are busy with their motor milestones, such as cruising, tipping lamps over, and getting their fingers pinched in doors, and they don't have time to talk. They put all their energy into getting places. Some have older siblings who interpret for them, and they don't need to talk. However, most babies will coo by about one to two months and vocalize at around four months. Do make sure your baby hears well. Hearing and language development go hand-in-hand. If she can't hear words, she can't learn to say them.

Incidentally, one study found that the way you talk to your baby can make a difference in encouraging language. Talking "baby talk" (i.e., using short, simple sentences, exaggerated intonation, and higher pitch) helped babies learn words faster than speaking to them as if they were adults.

How do I know my baby is hearing properly?

Babies receive the BAERS (brainstem auditory evoked response) hearing test at birth. It is one of the screening tests newborns get before they come home from the hospital. Sometimes babies fail the first screening in one ear or another. But the test is usually repeated in a month, and most babies pass by then. But if you have concerns about your child's hearing, he may need to be retested. Your pediatrician will continue to monitor hearing at well-baby visits. In the unlikely case there is general hearing loss, the baby should be seen by an ear, nose, and throat specialist.

At home, you can notice whether your infant starts at the sudden sound of a door slamming or an ambulance siren— and whether he coos and laughs by three months. Between six and nine months, he should respond to his name when you call, and begin to understand "bye bye" and "no."

How can I tell whether my baby can see properly?

Children do not have perfect 20/20 vision until age three. When they're first born, babies just see shapes and the mother's face, which is why it's important to look at your baby, interact, and smile. Babies can see black-and-white objects and complex shapes with high contrast. At about two months of age they recognize color. You can generally expect your baby to start focusing accurately by two to three months and to follow a slow-moving object by three months.

How do I know if my baby's cognitive development is normal?

Cognitive development tracks language and ability to think, learn, reason, and problem solve. By the end of the first year, I want a sense that babies are beginning to understand how the world works. They "get it" that when somebody leaves the room you wave bye-bye, and that playing peek-a-boo is fun.

What are the Apgar test and other hospital screening tests for newborns?

Newborns receive a battery of screening tests at the hospital before they go home, such as the BAERS hearing test, a basic examination of the red reflex of the eyes (to rule out cataracts), a variety of blood tests for conditions such as sickle cell anemia, cystic fibrosis, thyroid disease, and numerous metabolic disorders.

Perhaps the best known test is the Apgar score, a scoring system developed by Virginia Apgar that assesses color, tone, respiratory effort, heart rate, and reflex irritability after the baby emerges from the womb. Two points are awarded for each of the criteria, and a perfect score is ten. No baby should get a ten because all newborns have blue hands and feet. Circulation to the extremities takes a little time to get going. High scores suggest your baby got off to a roaring start. A low score can mean that the baby needs some medical intervention initially. Ask your doctor to interpret the score for you, but these early scores are not important.

The Apgar scores are given at one minute and five minutes after birth. Neither of these scores are predictors for later development. Many babies have a rough start, but are off and running at ten minutes. However, there is concern if the baby is still floppy, not breathing, and has a low heart rate at fifteen minutes. An Apgar score of two means the baby is in trouble. Continued difficulties after fifteen minutes may be predictive of neurological and cognitive problems ahead, but this should be discussed with the doctor.

Well-baby Visits

Regular well-baby exams at the pediatrician's office can detect potential health issues early and often prevent problems. The first visit usually takes place within forty-eight hours after the newborn leaves the hospital nursery, and then at two weeks, one month, two months, four months, six months, nine months, and twelve months. Every well-baby visit at my office covers feeding, elimination, sleep, growth, and development, along with any concerns or questions parents have.

As the baby grows, I assess three parameters by age: gross motor (rolling over, walking), fine motor (pincer, transferring an object from one hand to another), and language and social skills. The latter involve milestones such as smiling, interacting, deciphering language, and understanding cause and effect. There are many nuances in each of these areas.

Is it confusing for the baby if we use another language at home?

Babies learn language easily, and I applaud multilingual families. Studies suggest no delay in language in these households. My experience is that babies learn to understand different languages quickly but may be a little slower to speak.

What should I do if my baby's skills seem delayed?

Again, your pediatrician is your ally in evaluating progress and deciding whether another specialist needs to assess your baby. Government-funded Early Intervention programs are free for children under three years old. These programs can offer speech therapy, occupational therapy, and physical therapy.

Talking Together

Over the years, I've noticed that some parents have what I call a "report card mentality" about development that can stir a great deal of stress and interfere with the parent-baby relationship. They expect their child to start achieving at birth, sometimes even starting with the Apgar score. If their baby doesn't pass milestones early and get an "A" every time, mom and dad are distraught. Beware of this trap and talk together about expectations for your child. Clarify the wide ranges of normal with your spouse, and try to hang on to your perspective. Albert Einstein was a very late talker and also reputedly had an oddly shaped head as a baby.

An important question to explore together is "Can we allow our child to be himself and follow his own talents and interests? Or does he have to go to Harvard (or be an Olympic athlete or a concert pianist)? What if he's not an early reader?" Conversely, it's important to get your child assessed if a delay is worrisome. Both of you should discuss this with your pediatrician.

Of course we all want the best for our children, but every couple has different hopes and dreams. Realize that our children (like ourselves) are at least partially at the mercy of the genes passed on to them and circumstance. The perfect child doesn't exist. In fifth grade, nobody will care when he started crawling.

YOUR BABY IS UNIQUE

Parents often compare their child's growth and development with that of other babies, which can lead to needless anxiety. Instead, focus on the big picture and avoid jumping to conclusions, as many parents do. Pediatricians look at the overall development of your baby. It's the failure to do lots of different things at certain times that raises alarms. Progress is the key. Rely on your pediatrician to monitor your baby, and communicate your observations and concerns freely with her. If the doctor is satisfied, why not give yourself a break and revel in all the incredible changes in your baby so far.

CHAPTER 7

Babies' Bodies— From Head to Toe

This chapter covers:

- Head and scalp
- Eyes, ears, nose, and mouth
- Ancestry and babies' bodies
- Trunk and genitals
- Skin
- Hands and feet

Most new parents I see are enraptured by (and endlessly curious about) their baby. You, too, probably watch the baby sleep, listen to the baby breathe, and examine the baby's body every chance you get. Sometimes you may see a spot that wasn't there yesterday or notice a change that worries you, and wonder whether it's an abnormality or the baby could be sick. Most of the time it's something perfectly normal. Yet it's important to pay attention and ask your pediatrician about these concerns. You know your baby best, and you're an early warning system for the doctor.

Here are the common questions I hear from parents about their babies' bodies. The answers will help allay unnecessary fears you may have, and also alert you when your child should be seen by the doctor.

HEAD AND SCALP

I'm afraid I'll I hurt my baby's soft spot. How fragile is it?
The "soft spot" or fontanel often scares parents, but it is not as fragile as it looks. It is covered with a very tough membrane that protects the brain underneath, unless you inflict

a direct blow. In all my years of practice, I've never seen injury to the fontanel. The fontanel will close in the first year or two as the bones in the skull fuse together.

My baby has a crusty scalp. Why, and what can I do about it?

This is probably a form of seborrheic dermatitis (also known as cradle cap), which may appear in the first month of life. Babies usually outgrow it by their first birthday. To remove the crust, apply baby oil, corn oil, or olive oil to the scalp and gently massage it in to loosen the plaque. Wash out the oil with baby shampoo, and use a soft brush to very gently remove the scales.

I feel a lump on the back of my baby's head. Could he have hit his head without my knowledge or could it be a tumor?

Often the lump is just part of the baby's skull, which is sometimes asymmetrical. Ask your doctor about it. If it is a bony prominence or part of the skull, you can ignore the lump. If your baby hit his head, you would probably know it unless someone else was taking care of him at the time. Bumps on the head from trauma are usually firm, may look like a bruise, and can be tender to touch. Other bumps or lumps, such as certain benign cysts, can appear on the head from birth.

A lump located behind the ear or in the neck area might be an enlarged lymph node. Lymph nodes are collections of white blood cells that can cause swelling in response to an infection or inflammation nearby, such as cradle cap. Your doctor can help sort out what the lump is.

My daughter's soft spot seems to pulsate. Is that a problem?

No. These are normal arterial pulsations that you can sometimes feel in the soft spot. On the other hand, a depressed or indented fontanel may indicate dehydration. A bulging fontanel in a sick baby can be a sign of meningitis or increased pressure inside the skull. These diagnoses must be made by your pediatrician.

My baby has a cone head after delivery. Why does this occur and how long will it take before he has a normal head shape?

The cone shape is very common right after birth, especially in premature babies. In order to fit through the birth canal, babies' heads are molded into a shape that allows passage. Babies delivered by Caesarean section have perfectly round heads because they skip the journey through the birth canal. A cone-shaped head will remodel itself and become round in a few months.

How can I prevent my baby from developing a flat head?

This is an example of the law of unintended consequences. The incidence of positional plagiocephaly (a flattening of one side of the head) has increased dramatically since it became known in the early 1990s that sleeping on the back may help prevent SIDS deaths. A flat head occurs because the baby lies in one position all the time—often resuming the position held while in utero for nine months. You can prevent flattening beginning at about one month of age. Place the baby on her tummy for a few minutes each day (under supervision) while she is awake. This gets her off the back of her head. Because most babies do prefer to rest their heads on one particular spot, you can also turn her around in the crib to allow her to look at the other side of the room. You might put a picture on the wall or a stuffed animal on a shelf in the line of vision to give her something to look at and accustom her to this new position.

A flat head is a temporary problem. Eventually, the head will remodel into a normal shape, although it's a slow process that may take months to years to resolve because bone is being reshaped. Helmets were in vogue several years ago to prevent or help remodel a flat head, but they are now thought to be unnecessary in most cases and are rarely used.

Why is my baby losing his hair? Is something wrong?

Many babies lose their hair after birth, and some temporarily develop male pattern baldness, often resembling the father's. Don't worry about it because the hair eventually grows back. The bald spot from lying on his back will also eventually go away.

Why does my baby have so much hair?

Hair color and quantity and quality of hair are determined by the genetic mix the baby inherits from both parents. I often tell parents to look at baby pictures of themselves or other family members. Frequently mom and/or dad's hair in infancy was similar to the baby's.

Will my baby's hair color change?

Hair color can certainly change and often does. If your baby is blonde, and you and your spouse both have dark hair, there's no need to get a judge. Just wait a few months and the baby is likely to be brunette just like you.

EYES AND EARS

My baby has red marks on his eyelid. What are they and will they go away?

These are tiny capillaries or blood vessels, which are sometimes called stork bites or *nevus flammens*. They may also appear in the center of the forehead and the nape of the neck. The marks are most noticeable in Caucasian babies, especially those that are very fair skinned. As time goes by and the baby grows, these marks will become less noticeable.

My baby's eyelids and eyebrows are flaky. Should I apply a cream?

This is a form of seborrhea dermatitis, which babies usually outgrow by one year. Apply a good moisturizer like Eucerin cream or Aquaphor to lids and brows to keep them moist.

When my baby wakes up from a nap, her eyes seem to be swollen. Why does this happen?

Edema or fluid can accumulate around the eyes in the first few weeks of life. You're likely to notice it when the baby wakes after lying in one position. Don't worry about it unless the swelling remains after the baby is upright for a while.

My baby seems to be cross-eyed. Will this last?

Cross-eyes are known as "strabismus." Newborns often cross their eyes, but it's usually temporary. We don't necessarily do anything about it unless the eyes still cross after two months of age. In that case, a visit to a pediatric ophthalmologist may be necessary. There is also a condition called pseudo strabismus, which looks like cross-eyes, but is not. This is actually an illusion created by babies' wide nasal bridges. Your doctor can do a simple test in the office to determine whether the strabismus is pseudo or real.

If you notice one eye consistently turns in or out, bring it to the attention of your pediatrician. Treatment varies from watchful waiting to patching the eye, prescribing eyeglasses, or performing surgery. The point is to avoid the possibility that one eye will not be used enough.

One of my baby's eyes seems to be bigger than the other. Should I be concerned?

In some babies, the orbit of the eye or the eye socket is asymmetric in shape, which is not abnormal. Sometimes one pupil is bigger than the other from birth (known as anisocoria). Anisocoria does not affect vision, but it's important to know whether your child has this condition in case of a head injury later in life. When head trauma occurs, asymmetric pupils can be a sign of increased pressure on the brain from a bleed. Medical personnel must be told that the pupils are *normally* asymmetric and not a result of the head trauma.

Will my infant's eyes stay blue?

There is no way to know with certainty, although hazel, light blue, and green eyes are most likely to change color. Blue eye color is a recessive trait, which means the baby must receive the blue gene from both parents in order to have blue eyes. In contrast, brown eye color is dominant. If the baby gets two brown eye color genes from just one parent, he will probably have brown eyes.

There's a cut behind the bottom of my baby's ear that won't go away. What causes it, and what should I do about it?

This is another form of seborrheic dermatitis, which may be accompanied by flaking. If the cut opens, it can become infected. To prevent that, apply 0.5 to 1 percent hydrocortisone cream, which you can buy over the counter. Apply the cream three times a day until the cut is healed. If there is a discharge, ask your doctor to examine the baby.

My baby's ears have turned red. What's causing this?

Many times it's part of a nervous system response and is nothing to be concerned about. Some people have ears that turn red when they blush. However, it's worth investigating if the ears are red when the baby has a cold along with fever and irritability. Check with the doctor because it might be an ear infection.

NOSE AND MOUTH

Why does my baby sneeze so much? Does he have a cold?

Sneezing is a normal way for the body to rid itself of irritations and clear the nasal passage. Because babies cannot blow their noses, they sneeze. It may be a cold if sneezing is accompanied by severe nasal congestion, possibly a fever on the first day or two, decreased appetite, irritability, drowsiness, or possibly a cough. Usually babies develop a cold when someone else in the household has a cold.

My baby always sounds congested? What can I do about this?

It's normal for babies to make a certain amount of mucus. The only thing you can do is make sure air in the house is moisturized either with a pan of water on the floor or a cool mist humidifier (as long as you clean it). A bulb syringe can suck some mucus out of the nose unless it's lodged way in the back. Some medical professionals recommend putting a few drops of nasal saline in the nose to loosen up mucus before using the bulb syringe. I personally do not recommend drops because I find they make the baby cry, resulting in more mucus production. Do not use over-the-counter decongestants. They are not considered safe for children under six years of age.

My baby snores at night. Should I be concerned?

Snoring can either result from a nose blocked with mucus or from large adenoids, which are lymphoid tissues situated in the back of the nose area. Thirty or forty years ago, adenoids (and tonsils) were removed. Today we feel they are probably helpful in fighting infection. They also get smaller with age. They are occasionally removed for certain reasons, but not routinely. However, if the baby breathes through his mouth or wakes frequently at night due to the blocked nose, the adenoids are removed. If your baby snores every night, tell the doctor. Babies need high quality sleep, and some snoring babies don't get it.

My baby has a sore on her lip. What can this be?

This is probably a herpes simplex viral infection. Most of us are exposed to herpes type 1 at some point in early childhood, and recurrent outbreaks on the lip can occur. It could also be a sucking blister from breastfeeding if it's located in the middle of the lip. Occasionally, infants get sores, which can be an *aphthous stomatitis* viral infection inside the lip or mouth. There is no effective treatment for these sores in young babies. Keep her well-hydrated while the sore heals itself—usually in a few days.

I've noticed a white substance inside my baby's mouth. What is it?

It could be milk that's trapped on the surface of the tongue. To determine whether milk is simply coating the tongue, you can try to remove the milk with a piece of gauze or a soft toothbrush. If the milk doesn't come off—and there are white patches inside the cheeks or around the gums that won't come off either—the problem is likely to be a yeast infection called thrush. (See Chapter 2 for more information on causes of thrush.) Call the doctor.

When my infant cries, one side of his mouth seems to be lower than the other. Is this okay?

After delivery, there may be a temporary paralysis of the facial nerve that causes the mouth to look lopsided. One of the branches of the facial nerve may have been temporarily damaged during delivery. The condition should resolve within a few months. With the decrease in use of forceps at delivery, this condition is rarely seen.

How do I know if my baby has a tongue tie?

Underneath the tongue is a piece of tissue called the frenulum that attaches the tongue to the floor of the mouth. When this tissue is short and does not allow adequate tongue movement, it is called a tongue tie. Tongue ties used to be cut routinely, but the practice was probably overdone. Current practice is to cut it only when a baby has trouble sucking—or with enunciating words later on.

My baby seems to have a tooth in his gum, but my friends say he's too young to have teeth. If it's not a tooth, what is it?

Right after birth, babies can have "neonatal teeth," which are dangerous because they can be loose and may be swallowed. They should be removed. Often we also see little white bumps that can look like teeth and are called Epstein pearls. These are actually little cysts filled with epithelia or liner cells that are totally harmless and don't need any attention. Most babies don't get teeth until around four or five months of age, and sometimes much later than that.

My baby cries every time I try to give him a bottle. What could cause this?

Sometimes babies are just not hungry, or the hole in the nipple is too small and he is frustrated that the milk flow is not coming out fast enough. The same thing can happen if a mother's milk supply is down, and the baby is hungry. But if this happens consistently, see your doctor for a diagnosis. It could be colic, thrush, or a viral infection like Coxsackie virus.

How early do babies suck their thumbs, and is thumb sucking okay?

Some suck their thumbs in utero. Others discover their thumbs later. Sucking is a normal need for a baby.

Ancestry and Babies' Bodies

Our American melting pot includes greater diversity today than ever before, and certain physiological differences associated with ancestry are often seen in babies. For example, a 2002 study in northern California found that Hispanic, Chinese, Asian Indian, or other Asian infants were shorter and had lower birth weights and head circumferences than Caucasian babies. Pediatricians take such differences into account when evaluating babies' progress.

Often Asian (and some European) babies have hyperpigmented areas called Mongolian spots that look like bruises. These are simply areas of increased pigmentation that are harmless. They can be anywhere but usually appear on the lower back or buttocks. It's important to know about Mongolian spots to head off misunderstandings. One unfortunate family whose baby had this pigmentation was unfairly accused of child abuse.

Over half of baby boys in the United States are circumcised, although percentages vary with the region. The Midwest has the highest percentage of circumcised babies; the West has the lowest percentage. It is traditional for Jewish and Muslim male babies to be circumcised.

TRUNK AND GENITALS

What is the indentation I see in my baby's chest?

Pectus excavatum, which is Latin for "concave chest," is a common variation of normal that occurs in 1 out of 300 or 400 births. The concavity usually occurs right before the tip of the sternum or chest bone. Forget about it unless the curve is so severe that it compromises respiration (which is extremely rare). Although the curve is permanent, it becomes less noticeable as the baby grows into his body. If you go to the beach, you'll notice some adults who have this curve. Surgery is possible for purely cosmetic reasons. There is no evidence surgery improves cardio-respiratory function, except in extreme circumstances.

Why does my baby have a red spot on his chest that seems to be getting bigger?

This is probably a hemangioma, a group of blood vessels that usually start out as a flat vascular or red mark at birth and then becomes lumpy. A hemangioma is a common vascular anomaly that usually grows larger and more swollen. However, it should shrink back to its size at birth by the time your child reaches age three or four. Hemangiomas can appear anywhere, and only need to be treated when they block vision, compromise breathing or eating (as when located inside the mouth), or cause a serious cosmetic problem. If hemangiomas remain large, they can be treated by laser which will gradually shrink the lesion.

Sometimes when I watch my baby breathing, I notice a bump in the middle of his abdomen. What is it?

This is a kind of hernia called a ventral hernia, which is a weakness in the abdominal wall. It usually closes on its own and is not harmful.

I've noticed a brown spot under my baby's nipple? What is it?

If it falls in the nipple line, it may be an "accessory nipple," which is an extra nipple that is harmless. Nothing needs to be done about it.

Why does my baby seem to have breasts?

After birth, estrogen hormones that both girls and boys receive from the mother occasionally stimulate the breast.

Some milk production, called witch's milk, may even occur. Usually the breast enlargement disappears in a few weeks or so. Similarly estrogen may cause some labial and vulvar swelling in girls, which usually goes away within weeks. Baby girls occasionally have a mini-period with vaginal bleeding, which only lasts a day or two.

Why does my baby's belly button stick out?
It's the luck of the draw after the umbilical cord falls off. Pronounced "outie" belly buttons can be associated with an umbilical hernia, which is a little opening in the abdominal wall. As the baby grows and is able to increase abdominal pressure by crying or bearing down, you may see a more prominent belly button because a loop of bowel is pushed through that hole if it's big enough. This can alarm you, but the umbilical hernia usually closes by itself.

Why is there a little rubbery fleshy bump on my baby's umbilical stump?
Some babies develop granulomas, small amounts of extra tissue. These are harmless, but can be cauterized for cosmetic reasons with a silver nitrate stick in the doctor's office. The granulomas will turn gray or black and eventually disappear.

Why is there a lump in the baby's groin area?
This should be checked by a pediatrician. It could be enlarged lymph nodes due to something as simple as diaper rash. But it could also be an inguinal hernia, a weakness in the soft tissue around the groin area that causes swelling. This hernia needs to be evaluated. A hernia can also cause enlargement of the scrotum.

Why is my baby's scrotum so swollen?
After birth, many boys have extra fluid in the testicular area, called hydrocoele. The fluid is gradually reabsorbed by the

body and the scrotum returns to normal size. Your doctor can make this diagnosis by shining a light through the scrotum. If the light goes through, the swelling is caused by extra fluid.

My circumcised baby has a lot of extra skin on his penis, as though he hasn't been circumcised. Why?

Occasionally circumcision can leave redundant foreskin in place. If parents are unhappy with this redundant skin, I usually recommend a consultation with a pediatric surgeon for a redo (which is mainly for cosmetic reasons). The baby is circumcised, but the result is not perfect.

Sometimes I can't feel one of my baby's testes. What does this mean?

During fetal development, the testes gradually follow a passage from the abdomen to reside in the scrotum. Occasionally, one or both testes do not complete the journey. They are undescended and remain in the abdominal wall. Undescended testes must be corrected surgically by age three because they put the child at risk for cancer later in life.

More commonly, male babies have "retractile testes," which tend to move up from the scrotum to reside in the fat right above the scrotum. These babies have an active cremasteric reflex, which causes the testes to move up out of the scrotum in response to a stimulus such as cold. This reflex is normal, and as long as the testes can easily be brought down to the scrotum by your doctor, there is no concern. Eventually, the testes will reside in the scrotum where they belong.

Any time I change the baby's diaper, he seems to want to touch himself. Should I be concerned?

No. Self-exploration of genitals is very normal. There is no reason to be anxious about it.

Why is mucus coming out of my daughter's vagina?

An effect from the mother's estrogen may cause some mucus production in the baby for a short time. It's perfectly normal and there's no reason to do anything except clean it with warm water after a dirty diaper.

My friend's baby had a dislocated hip. How can I be sure my baby's hip is in place?

Your pediatrician will examine for signs of this at well-baby visits and perform certain maneuvers to check whether the hip is in place. Because there is a strong genetic component, you should let the doctor know if there is a family history of dislocated hips. You can also check for a dislocated hip your-self. When you turn the baby onto her stomach, look at cer-tain creases called the gluteal creases, which fall below each buttock. The creases should be symmetrical on both sides. If not, it could be a sign of a dislocated hip. Bring it to your pediatrician's attention. These babies may need to be seen by an orthopedist for triple diaper treatment (three diapers holding the hips in proper position) or some sort of harness.

My baby has a little tuft of hair and a dimple just above his buttocks. Is this a problem?

Three percent of normal babies have the dimple, which is known as a sacral or pilonidal dimple. This is present from birth and usually innocuous. The dimple is a small pit or hollow area at the top of the crease between the buttocks (known as the sacral area). Tufts of hair may also grow there. Because dimples can be associated with spinal cord abnormalities, your pediatrician will want to be sure the dimple is a closed pouch, rather than an open canal that could communicate with the spinal cord (a dangerous but rare occurrence). In such cases, lumbrosacral ultrasound may be required. If there is swelling or redness, check with your doctor.

SKIN

My baby has coffee-colored spots on his body. What are they?

Many babies have these spots, called café au lait spots. But you should be concerned only if six or more are present. In that case, the baby needs to be screened for neurofibromatosis, a genetic disease that presents in two forms. Type 1 affects 1 in 3000 people; type 2 affects 1 in 40,000. Early detection is important to permit screening for small growths called neurofibromas that grow along the nerves. Remember that a few of these spots is entirely normal.

My baby has a white spot on his body that is lighter than his skin. Why?

Hypo-pigmented spots can be many different things. Sometimes inflammation can cause loss of pigment in skin, which is common in babies with eczema. White spots can signify a fungal infection, which is rare in babies. A single white spot on the back can be a sign of tuberous sclerosis, which is very rare. In babies, however, white spots usually indicate prior inflammation. Eventually the pigment will return.

Why does my baby seem to have acne at one month? He isn't a teenager.

Maternal hormones start to drop off around three to four weeks of age. The drop-off may cause pimples on the face and upper chest. This acne lasts one to two weeks and does not need to be treated. If it extends beyond the neck and upper chest, call your doctor. It may not be acne.

Why does my baby seem to have whiteheads on his nose?

These "milia," are little blocked glands and are totally harmless. Eventually they disappear.

Why is my newborn's skin dry and peeling—like she's been sitting in the bath too long?

Many babies shed a layer of skin after birth, which usually does not require treatment. Post-term babies, delivered after their due date, are most likely to have dry, peeling skin. They have been sitting in the "bathtub" of amniotic fluid too long. If your baby continues to have dry skin, I recommend an unscented cream like Eucerin, Aquaphor, Lubriderm, or Moisturelle.

What are the most common birthmarks in babies?

Hemangiomas, compound nevi, café au lait, and salmon patches (also known as stork bites) are the most common birthmarks.

HANDS AND FEET

There's a straight line across my baby's palm, which I've heard is called a simian crease. Does this mean my baby has Down syndrome?

Actually one out of thirty normal healthy people has a simian crease. It's nothing to worry about. Today most Down's babies—who have bilateral simian creases—are diagnosed prenatally through ultrasound and sophisticated prenatal care. Down syndrome babies have other characteristics in addition to a simian crease. Pediatricians and nursery personnel are trained to look for these signs.

One of my baby's toes on each foot seems to turn in. Is this a defect?

It's a common variation of normal called clinodactyly, which is a descriptive term for "toe turning in." This is an inherited trait and usually is not a problem.

Why do my baby's legs turn in?

The position of babies' feet and legs in the first few months usually results from their position in utero. It takes a while to straighten out. The entire leg may turn in or out (called femoral anteversion or exoversion) or the knee down may turn in (called tibial torsion). Sometimes both legs turn the same way (called windswept feet). Turned-in feet alone, which is most common, is called metatarsus adductus. Years ago, bars and reverse shoes were used to correct these conditions. Today, treatment is usually not necessary because the result is the same—normal lower extremities whether you treat or not. Rarely, a turned foot is due to a structural

Talking Together

You and your spouse each bring expectations about your new baby to the table, and it's important to discuss them. For example, how important is your child's appearance to you? Not every baby is a knockout. What if she isn't perfect or cute or beautiful? She might even be a little homely. Maybe your son is going to be very short and won't be a basketball player. You're mixing two gene pools, and your baby may be very chubby or have a big nose, a receding chin, or freckles. Is this going to affect your feelings toward your child? Talk together about how to deal with disappointment to head off any damage to your relationship with your baby.

We live in an era where physical perfection is expected. Chances are your baby will have physical quirks. Once you understand what these variations are, you can move on and enjoy your child.

anomaly, such as a club foot, which does need orthopedic treatment.

Why are some babies' toenails misshapen?
Dysmorphic nails are common in babies. Nails can look wrinkled and hard and even grow into the soft skin of the big toe. Usually they turn into healthy, smooth nails with time. Ingrown toenails may also occur in babies; occasionally they become inflamed and even infected. The big toe is usually involved. If it becomes red, swollen, and tender to the touch, be sure to see your doctor because occasionally the ingrown toenail becomes infected and needs antibiotic treatment.

A PROCESS OF DISCOVERY

In many ways your baby's body is a mystery that keeps unfolding. You will find that your child will outgrow certain conditions; others are permanent but harmless. Remember that most major physical anomalies are now detected before birth by ultrasound. Those that are not detected are usually found at birth.

Because you and your spouse are involved in the baby's daily care, you know the landscape of your child's body intimately. At the same time, there are many opportunities for you to examine your baby with the doctor and ask questions. If you have a concern, never hesitate to bring it up.

CHAPTER 8

Day-to-Day Baby Care—
The Basics

This chapter covers:
- Bathing
- Care of umbilical cord, fontanel, genitals, nails, ears, and teeth
- Babies and pets
- Baby's comfort indoors and outdoors
- Choosing a pediatrician
- Babyproofing your home
- Traveling with baby
- Technology and your baby

A baby lights up your life, yet is also high maintenance. Part of everyday routine is keeping your child comfortable, clean, protected, and in harmony with the family as a whole. It takes time and effort, and there's so much to learn. These questions will help you sort out the challenges and arm you with information to start your new life with baby:

PERSONAL CARE

When should my baby take his first bath?
As soon as the umbilical cord falls off. This usually occurs within a few weeks of birth, although it can vary and take as long as a month. Until the cord separates, give him sponge baths. You want to keep the cord area dry.

How should I bathe the baby?
Bathe her either in the bathtub or in a small plastic tub you can put in a bathtub or sink. Many parents find it easier (and

a back saver) to get into the tub along with the baby. Always check water temperature before lowering her into the tub. Use mild unscented soap and be sure to keep a firm grip because babies can be slippery when soapy and wet. Never leave the baby alone in the tub, even for a second.

Do I have to use baby bath products all the time, rather than the same soaps, shampoos, and creams I use?

It's fine to use adult bath and hair products as long as they do not contain added perfume. (Adult shampoos tend to be very perfumed.) Only babies with extremely sensitive skin need to use special products. After a bath, moisturize the baby with an unscented moisturizer such as Aquaphor or Eucerin.

Should I use baby towels?

There is no reason to use special towels and wash cloths unless you want to. The towels in your home are fine. However, there are baby towels with a hood that make it easy to swaddle the baby after a bath on the way to the changing area.

How should I take care of the umbilical stump?

Years ago, alcohol was used to keep the umbilical stump clean. Studies have shown warm water will suffice, followed by exposure to the air. Fold the diaper down to keep urine from touching the stump. You want that cord to dry out and fall off.

How do I know if the cord becomes infected?

Keep an eye out for signs of infection, such as redness around the stump, a pus discharge from the cord, and possibly a foul odor. The baby may also have fever. If these symptoms are present, call your pediatrician, who may prescribe an oral or topical antibiotic.

The umbilical stump fell off and is bleeding. What should I do?

Bleeding is normal and will stop on its own. Just clean up the blood and apply pressure.

My baby is not circumcised. How do I take care of his penis?

Initially, there's nothing to do except keep the penis clean with warm water. As he gets older, his foreskin should be more and more retractable. Gently pull it back for very light cleaning.

My baby is circumcised. How should I care for the penis?

Right after circumcision, use gauze and petroleum jelly on the site. Primary healing usually occurs within a day or two, although the area may look raw or red. A dressing is no longer necessary after forty-eight hours. Watch for signs of infection, which is a possibility following any surgical procedure. However, I have never seen an infection develop from circumcision in my years of practice.

How should I clean my daughter's vaginal area?

Use warm water and a very soft wipe (no soap), but do not be overly vigorous or the vagina can become irritated. Just rinse off any stool near the area.

How should I care for the fontanel?

Nothing needs to be done for the fontanel.

I'm afraid to cut my baby's fingernails. Can I just leave them alone?

Babies often scratch themselves on the face or elsewhere unless their nails are cut. Many parents are afraid to trim, but it's important. Just use a gentle nail file or safety scissors.

Do not bite your baby's nails (as some parents do) because our mouths are filled with bacteria that can cause infection if the baby has a cut.

How about toenails?
Follow the same procedure as for fingernails.

I'm worried that my baby has an ingrown toenail. How do I know for sure and how is it treated?
Occasionally a baby's toenail will grow right into the toe itself. If the toe gets infected, it becomes red, swollen, and painful. Your pediatrician should see it. Most of the time, the nail will grow out on its own, but occasionally an antibiotic is prescribed.

Should I clean my baby's ears? If so, how?
Clean the exterior of the ear only, using a face cloth moistened with warm water. Any wax in the ear will eventually work its way out. Wax removal with a cotton swab can wind up pushing the wax further in, making it more difficult for your pediatrician later if he has to look at the eardrum.

My baby seems to be very itchy. How can I stop her from scratching?
Again, keep her nails trimmed to prevent scratching. But it's also important to know why she's so itchy. Most likely it's due to dry skin. If so, moisturize with an unscented moisturizer.

Is it okay to pierce my baby's ears?
Some cultures do this routinely—to both boys and girls, depending on the tradition. I have rarely seen a problem with ear piercing in infants but recommend waiting until after eight weeks of age. Some pediatricians pierce ears, but most parents have the procedure done safely in a retail setting. Make sure the place is very clean and is experienced

Babies and Pets

I confess. I love animals and am biased toward pets in the family. My husband and I always had two dogs that were like our children before our babies were born. After I became pregnant, we were very worried about the dogs adjusting to the baby. If you already have an animal, allow it to become accustomed to the new addition to the household. For example, we let our dogs sniff the baby, check her out, and be part of the family. But we would never leave a dog alone with her.

If you're about to get a dog, be sure to pick a breed that is relaxed around children. (Parents who already have a pit bull may have to give it up.) Labrador retrievers are great, and Portuguese water dogs are good with children, but most dogs, including mutts, are good family members. Some dogs are better choices if there is a family history of allergies. Labradoodles—a cross between a Labrador and a poodle—are among the dogs that shed less.

Cats are wonderful pets for children too, although they can be moody and are not as warm and loving as dogs. Cats also don't take well to mishandling by youngsters. You may want to have a pet cat declawed. There are short-haired cats that minimize the chances of causing allergies. As kids get older, cats can be good friends to them.

The best thing to do before acquiring any pet is to check with a veterinarian for suggestions. Animals are good for kids; they're fine companions. And when children grow up with pets, they learn to take care of someone else. They take on responsibility and are not just recipients of care. Fish and hamsters are wonderful choices, too.

with young ear lobes. If there is a pus discharge or odor around the earring, seek medical attention.

What should I do about teething?

Frozen bagels, frozen teething rings, or teething biscuits feel good on erupting gums and seem to relieve discomfort. Babies are often fussy, and parents may be too quick to attribute it to teething. If the gums are not swollen, the fussiness is probably from another cause. I prefer not to use pain medications such as acetaminophen or ibuprofen for teething unless there is gum swelling. Babies tend to be overmedicated for teething.

When should my child see a dentist?

The AAP recommends going to a dental home, an office where your baby's dental needs can be met, as soon as she gets teeth. Doctors used to wait until three years of age before recommending dental care, but today pediatric dentists can do more for preventive care earlier. Pediatric dentists, who specialize in children's teeth, are preferred because they usually enjoy working with children. Their offices are set up to entertain and distract children during the procedures. However, your family dentist may be terrific with youngsters.

WEATHER AND CLOTHING

How soon after coming home from the hospital can my baby go outside?

Fresh air is healthy for baby and parents. Babies can go outside any time after discharge from the hospital, provided weather conditions are not extreme. Most carriages have protection to block wind and rain. Of course use your judgment. If there's a howling wind and the temperature is five degrees, stay indoors.

On the other hand, do not take the baby to crowded places, whether indoors or out. The greatest threat to babies in the first eight weeks is infection.

What outdoor clothing should my baby wear?

Dress him according to the weather, using yourself as a guide. If it's too cold for you, it is too cold for the baby. When you're unsure, you can always feel his hands and feet. Layering clothing is always best because you can remove a sweater, for example, if it's warmer outside than you thought. You don't want the baby to overheat and catch a chill. However, remember he is not moving the way you are and may need an extra layer in cold weather. A hat is essential to retain body heat in the cold and shield him from the sun in warm temperatures.

Must I wash the baby's clothes separately?

There is no reason to wash her clothes separately unless she has extremely sensitive skin. Any detergent used for your own clothes is fine for your baby. Keep it simple. Life is hectic enough already.

When is the baby ready for shoes?

Babies need shoes to protect against foreign bodies and dirt, and for warmth—not for support. Once the baby starts walking, the best shoe is a soft flexible style that allows him to support himself. Because babies are clever at removing shoes and socks, choose shoes that foil attempts at removal. Hard shoes are expensive and unnecessary, and the cute little running shoes or ballet slippers you got at the baby shower probably won't stay on.

Should the baby wear sunglasses outside?

New recommendations from the AAP suggest that eye protection from ultraviolet rays is important for young eyes. We all should protect our eyes from sunlight. However, it may be a challenge to keep sunglasses on a baby whose little hands are busy.

Is it okay to use sunscreen on my baby?

Avoid too much sun exposure on the baby, especially between the hours of 10:00 a.m. and 2:00 p.m. But if the baby is going to be exposed, use baby sun block 30 SPF. Use hats, sunglasses, and clothes to cover him up. Babies under six months should stay out of direct sunlight.

When I walk my baby outside, should I talk to her?

Absolutely. This is an ideal time for you and the baby to talk to each other, which encourages language development. Make eye contact, smile, and point out, "See all the beautiful trees/squirrels/etc." You want to teach your baby to understand and use words. Put the cell phone away.

How to Choose (or Switch) a Pediatrician

Your baby's doctor is the single most important source of advice on your baby during the first year. Research suggests that pediatricians provide primary care services for most children (especially babies), and family practitioners see the rest. However, some care may be provided by nurse practitioners or physician's assistants who work with the doctor. A small percentage of pediatricians (less than 5 percent) known as "Med Peds" are trained in both family medicine and pediatrics. Personal referrals from friends, neighbors, and relatives are always best.

Consider these issues, too:

- Is the doctor covered by your health insurance? This will determine how much out-of-pocket cost you will have to absorb yourself.

- Is it a solo or group practice? Both have advantages and disadvantages.
- What is the doctor's hospital affiliation? Ideally your baby should go to a children's hospital where the staff are skilled at treating children. Often that isn't possible. But many hospital emergency rooms are staffed with doctors trained in both adult and pediatric medicine.
- Do you feel comfortable with the doctor? Remember this is one of the most important relationships in your life right now. If possible, meet and talk to the doctor before signing on. You can visit the office, interview the pediatrician, and get a feel for the office staff.
- How is the office run? "We had to wait two hours every time the baby went for a checkup," says one mom. "The office was chaos, full of screaming babies. I hated going there because it was such a stressful experience." Although every practice has its bad days, if that's the scenario all the time, you may want to go to a more efficiently run office. Because of the nature of medicine, however, there will always be unexpected delays for one reason or another.

If you don't feel a connection with the doctor or you're unhappy with the physician for other reasons, don't just settle. Trust is crucial. Perhaps you can switch to another doctor you like within a group, or ask neighbors, friends, or relatives for suggestions. You can also search the AAP and AAFP (American Academy of Family Physicians) Web sites for referrals in your area.

BABY'S ROOM

What's the proper temperature for my baby's room?

Many parents assume the baby's room should be hot. In fact, you can maintain the same temperature in your home that you normally do, unless you are an extreme energy saver, and the house is freezing. If the baby's hands are cold, cover them or add a layer of clothing. Take off a layer if the baby feels hot or is sweating.

Should I use a humidifier in the baby's room?

The cells that line the human respiratory tract flourish in a cool moist environment. Therefore, we all do better if the air is slightly moist. A humidifier works or simply place a pan of water on the floor. The water will evaporate and moisten the air. Humidifier filters should be cleaned regularly, and the pan of water changed periodically.

Babyproofing Your Home and Re-Proofing It

Part of your job is staying a step or two ahead of your baby, who can be amazingly resourceful and creative at getting into trouble as he develops new skills and explores.

- Clear the floors of items you're likely to trip on when carrying the baby in the middle of the night. Scatter rugs and toys lying around can be hazardous. Store toys in containers.
- Safety lock any storage location for toxic substances. Babies love cabinets under the sink in the kitchen and bathroom and are capable of eating cleaners and detergents or worse. Make sure medicine cabinets are out of reach.

- Check door locks to ensure a walking child can't accidentally lock himself in a room. Remove any locks that are potential hazards. One of my sons accidentally pushed in a door lock and we had to call the fire department to get him out.
- Keep the toilet lid covered (and latched if possible). We once returned home to find our daughter drinking out of the toilet while the babysitter napped. Babies do love toilets.
- Do not hang a picture, especially a low hanging one, over the changing table. Little hands can grab and pull it down.
- Beware of lamps a baby can pull down. Remove electrical cords and make sure window blind cords are out of the baby's reach.
- Place gates at the top and bottom of stairs. If you have a cat, gate off its own area to make sure the baby doesn't get into the cat litter.
- Double your safety awareness when you have visitors. As you concentrate on talking to a guest, it's all too easy for the baby to get into the person's handbag. This is one of the most common poisoning scenarios because people carry medications in their purses. Babies have eaten birth control or blood pressure pills.

See Chapter 11 for more hazards to watch. Unless you're superhuman, it's impossible to anticipate every possible danger to your child. Now and then accidents do happen. But if you stay alert, you can prevent most of them.

TRAVEL

When is my baby old enough to travel with us on an airplane?

Few people realize the risk of illness for young babies in airplanes, due to breathing recycled air with airborne viruses or touching surfaces covered with viral particles. Ideally wait until he's at least eight weeks old to travel. Babies are extra vulnerable to infections before that age because their immune systems are still immature. After two months, it's not such a big deal. People do travel with babies all the time. Some people bring wipes to clean around the seats, which is a good idea for all of us.

Note: Today, planes are pressurized and the effects on the ears are minimal. But you might want to consult your pediatrician if the baby had a recent ear infection.

What should we do if the baby won't stop crying on the plane?

Apologize to your neighbors and hope that the baby will soon fall asleep. This is one of those times where there's nothing much you can do.

What should I know about a car seat for my baby?

Whether you're driving your car to the supermarket or halfway across the country, make sure the baby sits in a properly installed child safety seat and is belted in. No newborn is allowed to leave the hospital without one. Proper use of these seats reduces deadly crash injuries to babies under one year by 71 percent, according to the National Highway Traffic and Safety Administration. (The seats reduce fatal injuries to children one to four years old by 54 percent.) The local police department usually will help you install a car seat in your vehicle. Babies under a year old and under twenty pounds should sit in a rear-facing safety seat, which is the safest position in case of collision. If you can, invest in a quality car seat. This is not the place to be frugal.

When purchasing baby equipment ranging from car seats to high chairs to strollers, look for certification by the Consumer Products Safety Commission and/or JPMA. You may also want to check out *Consumer Reports.*

How can we minimize the baby's crying in the car?

Babies are a hazard because there is nothing more distracting when you're driving than a screaming child. This is a time to either pull over or figure out what the issue is. People use food to distract babies old enough for something like a biscuit, or they play DVDs or music. Don't drive alone if you can help it. One couple schedules departure time for car trips according to when the baby is ready for a nap. He then sleeps for much of the journey.

When traveling try to maintain the same schedule the baby has at home; life will be much more pleasant. Expect the baby's sleep cycle to be disrupted in an unfamiliar place, and anticipate that it may take time to return to a routine when you get home.

How should I plan ahead for our vacation?

Consider whether the destination is baby friendly. Hotels may have resources you're not aware of; it's a good idea to inquire. Lots of better hotels have babysitters they've screened and cribs and play rooms, too. Get the name, address, and phone number of a pediatrician and a local hospital and emergency room in the area. You can go online or ask the hotel. If you're staying with friends or family, ask them. There are also many Web sites that offer advice on traveling with baby, such as the AAP site at www.aap.org.

When you visit friends or stay in a hotel, bear in mind it's up to you to childproof the area.

TECHNOLOGY AND BABIES

Is it okay for my baby to watch TV?

TV is very appealing, and it can be educational. The issue is what children are *not* doing while watching TV. They're not talking or interacting with a grown-up or being read to. Language and cognitive delays are linked to early TV viewing, yet 20 percent of babies have their own TV. A study has found 40 percent of three-month-olds watch TV, DVDs, or videos regularly. Research on 300 children ages two months to four years found youngsters heard 7 percent fewer words from an adult and talked less themselves for every hour the TV played. Television also has a role in children's obesity and consumption of junk food, and is linked to antisocial behavior.

I understand parents need downtime. After all, TV is a wonderful babysitter, and it is free. But be clear about why you're using TV, and realize it's seductive. Maybe you need to hire a babysitter instead. The American Academy of Pediatrics does not recommend TV for children under two years of age. It's also a bad idea to leave the TV on in the background while baby is around; the noise competes with the baby's focus on play or exploration.

How about videos that help make babies smarter?

There is now evidence that such well-marketed products do not aid babies' cognitive development and may even lead to smaller vocabularies.

Are any educational DVDs or videos good for babies?

Because most families turn the set on at some point, regardless of all the warnings, try to find videos that do not promote products, but that instead teach children numbers, letters, colors, and good behavior. Try to avoid hyperkinetic shows you may have grown up on, such as frantic cartoons.

Talking Together

Sit down and discuss how to prepare for hurdles that cause last-minute scrambles, such as a sick babysitter or the nanny's car trouble. Who needs to travel? Are there overnight nanny options if both of you are on business trips? Will grandparents fill in? Talk about who will go to well-baby visits. In some families, it's dad.

Negotiate sharing baby care tasks, and try to work out a fair division of labor. This is also a time to strategize problems like what to do about a pet now that the baby is here. One couple expected to ship their beloved dog to parents in another state, but the dog surprised them and was very good with the baby.

Map out strategies together about TV viewing or before you know it, your baby will be cooing at Barney and jiggling his head to all his favorite television friends for hours at a time. Most families let children watch TV some of the time, but be careful here. Talk, too, about when to introduce your child to the computer and what the downside may be, such as less physical and social playtime. On the other hand, technology does have advantages. Web cams allow babies and grandparents who live far away from each other to "visit" on a regular basis.

Concerns about technology include children's dependency on external stimuli and your modeling behavior if you can't put down your BlackBerry. You won't believe how quickly your baby may be grabbing for your cell phone, manipulating the TV remote, and erasing work on your laptop.

Music, soft tones, and repetition of the basics are best for little ones.

ENJOY YOUR BABY EVERY DAY

Day in and day out, you're building a new life with baby. It may seem strange and overwhelming at times, but you're going to be surprised at how quickly your confidence can grow and how issues that loomed large at first become routine. Try to savor and make the most of your daily experiences with your child. Today many mothers and fathers walk down the street with their babies while talking on cell phones. They're not interacting with the infant nor providing the kind of attention babies thrive on. There is growing evidence that the more language babies hear (from adults, not TV), the better they acquire speech and comprehension. Your words and interactions with your child benefit you, as well, adding pleasure and connection to your relationship.

CHAPTER 9

Immunizations—Facts and Fiction

This chapter covers:

- Vaccine basics
- First year immunization schedule
- Autism and vaccines
- Other immunization concerns

In the last thirty years, I've seen vaccines save children from the deadly effects of bacteria, such as Haemophilus influenzae and Streptococcus pneumoniae. Anti-viral vaccines against polio eradicated this scourge in the United States in 1978. We never hear of smallpox or diphtheria, as a result of vaccines. And inoculations have slashed the incidence of meningitis, pneumonia, and sepsis (blood infections), which killed so many children years ago. Despite these and other success stories, controversy continues to surround some vaccines. Following are the most common questions new parents ask me about immunizations. The answers will help clarify any confusion about the shots your baby needs—and their safety. Maybe someday we will be able to eliminate some of these vaccinations, as we have in the case of smallpox, where the disease has been eradicated from entire continents. In the meantime, the vaccines we have are saving children's lives.

UNDERSTANDING IMMUNIZATIONS

How do vaccinations help my baby?

Vaccines help protect against viral or bacterial infections that would otherwise harm children. Vaccines are effective because inoculating most children creates a phenomenon called herd immunity that makes it difficult for an infection to gain a foothold in the community. The more members of the "herd" who are protected, the less likely anyone will fall ill.

Not so long ago, serious bacterial infections such as epiglottitis (an infection of the upper airway), mastoiditis (an infection behind the ear), and meningitis (an infection of the lining of the brain and spinal cord) kept pediatricians awake all night. But life-threatening complications from ear infections or pneumonia are less likely now due to vaccinations. These complications are rarely seen today, a change that allows doctors to treat more minor infections less aggressively. For example, antibiotics were once thought absolutely necessary to treat ear infections to prevent complications such as mastoiditis. Widespread antibiotic use contributed to the rise of drug-resistant bacteria, a problem we face today. In response to antibiotics, organisms mutated, and treatment drugs were rendered less effective. But with incidents of mastoiditis becoming more rare, scientists now feel that watchful waiting and pain management is all that is needed to treat ear infections in certain situations..

Your baby will personally benefit from the protection vaccines provide. But along with the benefit comes parents' obligation to be good citizens by immunizing their children. Those who don't participate may jeopardize other children's health. If enough members of the "herd" go unvaccinated, the herd effect is lost, and more children become vulnerable to infection.

How do vaccines work?

Vaccines contain modified versions of the intended bacteria or virus that causes a certain disease. Sometimes the bacteria is inactivated or killed, as in the polio shot. Another type of vaccine uses only part of the bacteria to induce an immune response, such as the pertussis (whooping cough) or HIB vaccine (Haemophilus influenzae). "Live" vaccines contain attenuated or weakened versions of an organism.

Varicella (chicken pox) and the MMR (measles, mumps, and rubella) are live vaccines. The weakened organism stimulates the immune system to respond by making antibodies that fight the invading microbe. As a result, antibodies are already in place to attack if the bacteria or virus invades the body. Some vaccines such as the influenza vaccine come in both live and killed versions. Your doctor will suggest which one is right for your baby.

Why are some vaccines combined in one shot?
There are so many vaccines today that medical science tries to minimize the number of shots. Vaccinations are painful for babies, and fewer inoculations are more convenient for parents and doctors, as well. The newest combination is the Pentacel, which includes DTaP, or diphtheria, tetanus, and acellular pertussis; IPV, which is inactivated polio vaccine; and HIB, or haemophilus influenzae type-B.

Recommended Immunizations in Babies' First Year

This is the current lineup of vaccinations for the first twelve months. The list is subject to change because new vaccines are constantly added, and existing vaccines often become available in combination shots.

- Pentacel
- Hepatitis B (HepB)
- Hemophilus influenza type B (HIB)
- Rotavirus (RV)
- Pneumococcal (PCV7)
- Influenza
- Measles, Mumps, Rubella (MMR): First dose at a minimum of twelve months

---

- Varicella (chicken pox): Minimum age twelve months
- Hepatitis A (HepA): Minimum age twelve months

We no longer routinely test children for tuberculosis in the United States unless they've been exposed to an active case of the disease. Testing is done in localities with large immigrant populations from countries where TB is endemic. These nations may inoculate with BCG (Bacillus Calmette-Guerin) vaccine for TB.

Immunization Schedule

Note that timing of vaccinations can vary from community to community. Below is the schedule followed in my office in Boston. As you can see, some vaccines require more than one shot.

- At birth: HepB
- Two months: Pentacel, PCV7 (pneumococcal), HepB, Rotavirus
- Four months: Pentacel, PCV7, Rotavirus
- Six months: Pentacel, PCV7, HepB, Rotavirus
- Twelve months: PCV7, HIB
- MMR and varicella immunizations are given at anywhere from twelve to fifteen months. Hepatitis A is given at one year or older and requires two doses at least six months apart.

The influenza vaccine was once reserved for children at risk for complications of the flu. These were children with chronic conditions such as asthma, cancer, or autoimmune disorders. Today, all children over six months of age should get an annual flu shot in the fall. In 2009, the H1N1 vaccine was also recommended for all children over the age of six months.

Why are vaccines given at different ages?

Most vaccines for babies are given in a stepwise fashion to create and then boost immunity. The protection from just one shot is not enough. Inoculations are spread out over months, and then years, to create and enhance protection. Some vaccines, such as the MMR, cannot be given before twelve months because antibodies from the mother can cross the placenta, which stops the baby from making his own antibodies for the disease. When the mother's antibodies begin to wane, the baby will be unprotected.

Is it safe for the baby to be vaccinated when he has a cold?

Babies with mild upper respiratory infections can be vaccinated. These immunizations are important. The consensus is that it's better to give the shots as soon as possible to avoid the risk the child won't be inoculated at all. However, shots should be postponed in cases of high fever or severe illness.

Where does my baby get the shots?

We usually vaccinate in the upper outer thigh, where there is plenty of fat and muscle to absorb the impact of the shot.

What reactions should I expect to see in my baby after vaccination?

There may be mild and temporary side effects in some children. Your baby may fuss immediately because the injection hurts. Later, in the evening, she may cry because her leg is sore. Check to see if there is swelling or redness around the injection site; a cold pack can alleviate the swelling. Vaccinations can also cause fever lasting up to forty-eight hours. You can give her Infant acetaminophen drops (Tylenol)—or Children's ibuprofen (Motrin) after six months of age for pain or fever. Be sure to ask your doctor about appropriate dosage, which varies depending on your baby's weight. MMR vaccination can have a delayed reaction, including a rash and fever that usually occur a week to ten days later. The rash looks like a fine red spotty sprinkling on the trunk. There is no need to treat it. Call the doctor if fever lasts more than forty-eight hours or if the baby looks ill.

I have a very hard time watching my baby being vaccinated. What should I do?

This is common with some parents. I've seen a few who have almost passed out. If you have a phobia about needles, it's important not to transmit your fear to your baby. Ask the nurse to take your place and sit in the waiting room until it's over if you cannot control your anxiety. Children look to their parents for clues about any threat involved in a situation. If your fear spills over to the baby, he may overreact. After the shots, expect a loud wail, followed by indignant crying that usually ends by the time you reach the car or walk home.

If we travel to another country where we're required to get inoculations, should the baby get the same shots we do?

It depends on which vaccines are involved. Babies under a year are unlikely to get travel vaccinations. However, hepatitis A vaccine can be given from twelve months on; yellow fever vaccine can be given after nine months. Ask your doctor what's necessary and safe.

Is it likely that current vaccine guidelines will change?

Yes. We constantly look for ways to combine vaccines in order to reduce the number of shots babies receive. But extensive studies must be conducted to make sure that combinations do not negate the general effectiveness of any single vaccine or produce unwanted side effects.

Will my baby need booster shots for vaccinations as he gets older?

The answer is yes in some cases. For example, chicken pox vaccine is given at a minimum of twelve months. Recently we found children were becoming susceptible to the virus years later. As a result, a booster dose has been added at age five. DPT, MMR, and polio vaccines also require boosters at age five. Some of these need to be boosted again at age twelve and then every ten years. Scientists continue to study the length of time immunity lasts for various vaccines.

Recently it was discovered that whooping cough (pertussis) is actually more prevalent in older children, adolescents, and adults than was previously thought. It appears that the pertussis vaccine also has waning immunity. As a result, a booster is now recommended at twelve years, and then every ten years, along with diphtheria and tetanus.

Do vaccines provide 100 percent protection?

Nothing is 100 percent. A few people will catch any disease despite being immunized, but hopefully they will get a milder version. Boosters are required to maintain immunity in some vaccines.

My baby is allergic to eggs. Are there any vaccines she should not get?

Because the flu vaccine may contain egg protein, anyone with an egg allergy should not receive the vaccine. The MMR vaccine also may contain egg protein, but allergists assert that it is safe to give the MMR to a baby allergic to eggs. You might want to discuss this with your doctor and remind him about the baby's egg allergy.

AUTISM AND VACCINES

Why is there controversy about vaccines and autism?
The prevalence of autism has increased in recent years. According to CDC estimates, an average of 1 in 110 children in the United States has an autism spectrum disorder (ASD), and many parents of autistic children and certain others have blamed vaccines as the cause. A flawed study linking the MMR vaccine to autism has since been discredited. Many studies since then have disproved any linkage between MMR vaccine and autism, but many people still worry about a connection.

Another flawed linkage is that of thimerosol and autism. Thimerosol was once used in vaccines as a mercury preservative. However, there is no scientific evidence of a link between thimerosol and autism. In addition, thimerosol has been removed from most vaccines by manufacturers since 2001. Despite the removal, the autism rate has continued to rise. Most likely the vaccines used by your pediatrician today are virtually thimerosol-free. Certain types of vaccines do still contain a trace of thimerosol. If you're concerned, ask your pediatrician about them.

Can the MMR vaccine cause autism?
Critics of vaccines also believe combinations of vaccines in one injection may overwhelm the immune system, causing autism. The combination measles, mumps, rubella shot has been targeted for blame, despite studies showing there is no cause and effect between the MMR vaccine and autism. Although MMR vaccination rates have dropped due to parental worry about an autism link, the incidence of autism has continued to rise. A recent court ruling in a case brought by families of autistic children found there was no link between the measles virus in MMR vaccine (or between thimerosol) and autism.

Each week brings a parent to my office with a fear about autism. Many parents have read articles or blogs online that are not reputable sources, but that tout a link between MMR or thimerosol and autism.

Can my baby get shots one at a time instead of in combination?

Yes, but there is no medical reason to subject babies to multiple, rather than combined shots—and no evidence to support the idea that one-at-a-time is safer. Nevertheless, some worried parents consider this a "hedge" against autism. The issue strikes an emotional note, and they do not want to put their child at what they perceive is a possible risk. I always respect parents' wishes, although my office no longer administers the MMR vaccine in separate doses as there is no evidence this is beneficial.

It seems every year there are more vaccines. Why are we turning our babies into pincushions?

Modern medicine is trying to eradicate more diseases and reduce illness. For example, rotavirus, a viral infection that can cause severe diarrhea in children, is responsible for 100,000 hospitalizations and 250 child deaths a year in the United States (611,000 children annually worldwide). Four out of ten American children will have a rotavirus infection before five years of age. A new oral vaccine for rotovirus is now available to prevent it and is considered safe.

OTHER ISSUES

Do immunizations cause SIDS?

This is another myth about vaccines. A 2004 review of studies by the Institute of Medicine at the National Academy of Sciences found no connection.

It's unlikely my baby will be exposed to hepatitis B so why do I have to vaccinate her?

A very large percentage of people in this country are carriers of this disease. It's an insidious disease that can be transmitted through food handled by a carrier or through sexual activity with a carrier (who may not be aware of his or her status). The idea is to protect children before they are exposed to carriers.

I've read that the companies that make the flu vaccine don't know what strain will be prevalent in a particular year. Why should I give my baby a shot that won't protect him?

Immunizing populations is not a perfect science, but manufacturers try to identify which strains are likely to hit North America in a given year before they prepare the vaccines. Because many people die or become severely ill from influenza, it is worth taking the chance that the vaccine will be helpful.

Can my baby get the disease from the vaccination itself?

Because vaccines include modified versions of the infecting organism, it is possible that your baby will get a mild version of the illness.

I've heard of people contracting Guillain-Barre syndrome after receiving flu vaccine. Is my baby at risk?

In 1976, swine flu vaccinations (for a different strain from the H1N1 of 2009) were associated with Guillain-Barre, which is an inflammation of the nerves causing muscle weakness (and occasionally paralysis). Most people eventually recover, although it can take months. According to the Centers for Disease Control and Prevention (CDC), research on other flu vaccines since then has shown no connection with Guillain-Barre, except for a study that suggested one out of a million people receiving vaccine might get the syndrome.

I don't plan on using day care for my baby or taking her to public places. Is it necessary to vaccinate my baby?

I understand that you intend to keep your baby away from large groups of people, but it's not at all clear that your baby will *never* be in a public place—or that it's healthy to isolate your baby either socially or medically after two months of age. Babies need to build some resistance to infections. Your child will be in public places as she gets older, goes to school, and lives her life.

My father is undergoing chemotherapy for cancer. Should my baby be vaccinated if she is going to be in contact with my father?

Live vaccines—the MMR, varicella (chicken pox), or live flu vaccine—shouldn't be given to babies who will be in contact with immune-compromised individuals. The latter includes chemotherapy patients, people on certain arthritis medications, post–bone marrow transplant patients, and others. The issue is that the vaccinated baby may secrete even attenuated versions of the live virus or bacteria, which could cause the disease in a person with a compromised immune system. This is another reason to vaccinate your baby today, before the issue of sick relatives comes up.

Is it okay for me to be vaccinated if I'm pregnant?

Live vaccines can be a problem in the first trimester. The danger may have been exaggerated, but it is best to check with your obstetrician.

Talking Together

Vaccinations can be an emotionally charged topic for parents for a number of reasons. Many people become upset when their baby is getting a shot. They may feel guilty that they are allowing their child to be hurt by a needle. On a deeper level, one or both parents may have a friend or relative or coworker with an autistic child. It's natural to fear, "Could it happen to us?" Try to discuss this issue with your spouse before you bring the baby in for his shots. Again and again, I feel the tension between uncertain couples and hear their arguments about whether or not the baby is going to be vaccinated, and if so, how. If you need more time to make a decision, ask your doctor for information to take home to discuss privately. The Resources section at the back of this book lists authoritative online sources for additional information. Also see Chapter 13 for how to identify a questionable source.

REWARD VERSUS RISK

Vaccines protect the public health and have truly changed the world for the better. Measles and chicken pox, which wreaked havoc on small bodies, used to be regarded as rites of childhood. Today these diseases rarely occur in the United States thanks to vaccinations. Flu vaccine for children over six months old is an important protection. According to the CDC, 36,000 Americans die of the flu annually, and 200,000 more are hospitalized.

Children cannot enter school in most of the United States unless they have received the necessary immunizations. Of course, nothing is without risk, and sometimes you have to weigh the pros and cons and take your chances. Scientists work on a daily basis to reduce the risk of harm.

CHAPTER 10

Illness—Is the Baby Sick?

This chapter covers:

- Fever and how to manage it
- Colds, coughs, respiratory conditions
- Medicine chest basics
- Ear infections
- Stomach bugs, roseola, and other medical issues
- When to call the doctor

Most new parents experience a spectrum of anxieties about the baby's health, and you're likely to have your share. You may start by obsessing about SIDS, and then move on to a variety of illnesses you've read (or heard) about. It's only natural. You're so attached to this child and so afraid that something out of your control might threaten the baby, whether it's a flu scare or a nasty rash that erupts from out of nowhere. Despite your best efforts to sanitize every item and every person who enters your home, the reality is your baby is likely to get sick sometime in the first year—probably more than once. The challenge is separating what is routine, such as a cold, from something that might be more serious.

In my day-to-day practice, I (and the wonderful staff I work with) constantly field calls about symptoms that have suddenly developed (or changed), and we decide whether we want to see the baby. At other times, I respond to parents' "What should I do if . . ." questions stemming from what they generally worry about and what they've heard about from the Internet, other parents, or the media. Here are common queries—and answers that arm you with information you need to ward off panic and build confidence.

FEVER

What is considered a fever in a baby?

A rectal reading of 100.4 degrees or more is considered a fever (abnormally high body temperature). This usually signals the immune system is fighting an infection or other assault. Most fevers are caused by viral infections.

What are the signs of fever in a baby?

Experienced mothers and fathers know that if the baby's skin feels hot to the touch, he may have a fever. But he could also be hot from overbundling or crying. Other symptoms and signs help to tell whether the baby is sick or just overheated. The baby may look very pale or flushed, or act listless or fussy. Loss of appetite, excess sleeping or wakefulness, diarrhea, vomiting, runny nose, or a cough may occur. If someone else in the household is sick, the baby is more likely to come down with the same illness. In the end, trust your gut and take the baby's temperature with a thermometer to confirm a fever.

What is the best thermometer to buy, and how should I take temperature?

We view illness in the first eight weeks of a baby's life differently from later months because very young infants are vulnerable. Their immune systems are immature, and it can be very hard to tell the difference between symptoms of a cold and a serious bacterial infection. As a result, we want to know an exact temperature in a child this age. Use a rectal thermometer, which is the most accurate.

After eight weeks, you can buy a less invasive thermometer such as a skin sensor you can run across the forehead or an ear thermometer. If you take an axillary (under the arm) temperature, add a degree to the reading. If using an ear thermometer, make sure you have a good seal in the

canal to prevent a false low reading. Do not use an oral thermometer for a baby or toddler.

What should I do if the baby does have fever?

Call the doctor immediately if the baby is less than two
months old and has a temperature of 100.4 degrees or
higher—or if the reading is 102 degrees or more in an older
baby. (Don't hesitate to call, too, any time you're worried
about how the baby looks, regardless of the temperature.)
You can give acetaminophen (Tylenol) to babies under six
months, and acetaminophen or ibuprofen (Motrin or Advil)
to a baby over six months old. Pediatric doses are based
on weight. Ask your pediatrician for a weight-based dosage
chart. Most pediatric medications come in liquid form, usually with a dropper you can put in the baby's mouth. Follow
immediately with a bottle or the breast to prevent the medication from being spit out.

What if the temperature is really high?

A temperature of 104 degrees or more can be alarming to
parents, but a simple virus can cause such a reading. Try to
get the fever down by immersing the baby up to the neck in
a lukewarm bath. Although a cold bath may seem more log-
ical, cold water causes shivering, which raises the body temperature. Lukewarm water, which lowers the fever slowly, is
more effective. (We no longer recommend an alcohol bath
because alcohol can be absorbed and is not safe.) It may be
easier on your back to get into the bath along with the baby.
Be sure the water is neither too hot nor too cold. Add warm
water if the baby shivers. After twenty minutes, retake the
temperature. Most of the time the fever will have dropped.
With a lower temperature, you will have a better sense of
how sick the baby is. Once the child is a little cooler, you
can give acetaminophen or ibuprofen (depending on the
baby's age) and call the doctor. The doctor will ask ques-

tions such as, "How long has she had the fever?" and "What other symptoms does she have?" The treatment of fever is for your baby's comfort. Fever itself is usually not harmful and is helpful to signify illness.

I heard it is helpful to alternate acetaminophen and ibuprofen. Do you agree?

There is no added benefit from alternating acetaminophen and ibuprofen. This is one of so many treatment ideas that haven't stood up to the test of respected research studies.

My neighbor's baby had a seizure from a fever. Why does this happen?

Approximately three to five percent of children nine months to five years of age experience a febrile seizure, which tends to occur when fever rises very quickly. These seizures are usually harmless, although they terrify parents, who may not even know their baby is sick. It's frightening to see your child suddenly jerking, twitching, or shaking. When I was a medical student and my own daughter had a seizure, I thought she was dying. I was so frightened that I ran to the emergency room in my nightgown. Babies are very tired afterward, which is one way to know whether a seizure has occurred.

What should I do if my baby has a febrile seizure?

First make sure her airway is clear. Turn her head slightly to the side to prevent choking if she vomits. If she already has vomit in her mouth or mucus blocks breathing, try to clear it out with your finger to keep the airway open. Watch her color to make sure she is not turning blue. If a seizure lasts more than a few minutes, call 911 for airway support on the way to the hospital.

Fortunately, most seizures are over in seconds, and the next step is to call your doctor. The doctor may want to see the baby to rule out other diagnoses, such as a virus or spinal meningitis if she hasn't been vaccinated. Seizures are also associated with a bacterial intestinal infection called shigella, often with bloody diarrhea or a seizure disorder. There's a long list of possibilities.

Some babies are genetically disposed to febrile seizures, which can run in families. Seizures may recur, leading some parents to overreact and try to prevent them by plying a baby with anti-fever drugs like acetaminophen. There is little evidence to support this practice. Children do usually outgrow seizures by about six years of age.

COLDS, COUGHS, RESPIRATORY ISSUES

How do I know if my baby has a cold?
Signs include nasal congestion, coughing or wheezing, possibly more sneezing than normal, and loss of appetite. He might also be particularly irritable or less active than normal. A cold is viral, and fever often develops in the first forty-eight hours of any viral illness.

How should I treat my baby's cold?
If she has a fever, you can give proper dosage of acetaminophen or ibuprofen based on the baby's weight. (Check with your doctor if you haven't already asked for a dosage chart.) Be aware that cold and cough medications are not safe for children under six years old.

Because babies can't blow their nose when they have a cold, they either sneeze out mucus or sometimes swallow enough mucus to gag and vomit. Spitting up mucus can be helpful, as this is one way for the baby to clear her airway. When a cold is present, the baby may be more comfortable sleeping slightly upright in an infant seat. She may also need extra fluids such as breast milk, formula, or sterile water.

How can I prevent the baby from catching my cold when I'm breastfeeding?

There's not much you can do except wash your hands often with soap and warm water. The evidence shows hand sanitizers alone will not protect against upper respiratory viral illnesses like a cold.

Can I prevent my baby from catching his older brother's cold?

This is very difficult to prevent especially if the sibling is a toddler who doesn't understand a cold is contagious. The best bet is to try to keep the sibling from touching, sneezing, or coughing on the baby. Keep washing the toddler's hands (and yours). Children do tend to get frequent viral infections in day care and preschool because they're exposed to so many other children. They touch their nose and eyes and catch a cold. It's not all bad because they build their immune systems. When they're older, they'll probably have better immunity to these infections.

What's the difference between viral and bacterial infections?

Bacterial infections are generally more serious, but less common, and are usually treated with antibiotics. Most of the illnesses we see in babies are viral infections, which we often don't treat because antibiotics don't work for viruses. Nevertheless, some parents feel better if the baby receives medication, and they may pressure the doctor for a prescription. However, most of today's parents are more educated to the risk of overprescribing antibiotics when they're not appropriate. On the other hand, if your pediatrician feels your baby does need an antibiotic, do follow the instructions. In the office setting we often don't know for certain whether it's a virus or bacterial. Lab tests are expensive and not always available on site. Most of the time we use clinical judgment based on a good history and physical exam and encourage parents to stay in close contact with us in case there is a change for the worse in the baby's condition. Watchful waiting can be the best medicine.

Some families resort to herbal remedies or natural products for these illnesses. However, most of these remedies are not subjected to double-blind controlled studies (which are the gold standards we use for medications). I usually don't feel comfortable prescribing these products. A recent example is a homeopathic nasal spray containing zinc that was taken off the market after some users seemed to permanently lose their sense of smell.

Essentials for Your Medicine Chest in the First Year

Acetaminophen (Tylenol)

Ibuprofen (Motrin or Advil)

Bulb syringe for cleaning out the nose

Vaseline

Diaper cream with zinc oxide

Hydrogen peroxide

Hydrocortisone cream—0.5 percent or 1 percent (Use only with doctor's permission.)

Antibiotic ointment

Gauze

Band-Aids

Sun block—30 SPF

Good moisturizers, such as Eucerin or Aquaphor

Safety scissors to trim toenails and fingernails

Sharp forceps to remove splinters

Infant toothbrush and infant toothpaste

My baby has had a cold for two weeks and the nasal mucus is green. Is this a sinus infection?

It once was believed that green or yellow mucus indicated a bacterial infection, but we now know that the color represents white blood cells that can be present in virus infections, as well. In fact, sinus infection was grossly overdiagnosed in years past and is a rare diagnosis today. If an upper respiratory infection lasts more than ten days, it is possible that the baby has developed a secondary bacterial sinus infection. The baby looks sick, and the diagnosis is based on medical judgment. If your doctor thinks the baby does have a secondary infection, she will prescribe antibiotics.

My baby has had a stuffy nose and a cough for two weeks. Could this be pneumonia?

A diagnosis of pneumonia, a serious lung infection, is usually made when the baby has rapid respiration, retractions where you see his ribs when he breathes, and a prolonged cough with fever for over forty-eight hours. Call the doctor if these parameters are present. Babies with pneumonia may also be irritable, have poor color, and lack appetite.

Note that distressed breathing from a lung infection sounds different from the rattling of mucus in the baby's chest, which occurs because babies don't clear mucus very well. Deciphering which is which is a job for the doctor.

Last night I thought I heard the baby wheezing. What could it be?

Wheezing is often seen in young babies. It's commonly caused by bronchiolitis, inflammation of a small airway usually due to a viral infection. Wheezing tends to accompany a cold.

If there is a family history of asthma, eczema, or other allergies, it's possible that a wheezing baby is showing the first signs of future asthma. However unless the wheezing becomes an every night occurrence, it's unlikely an asthma diagnosis would be made in the first year. There is no test for asthma in babies.

My six-month-old nephew has something called RSV. He wheezes and seems to have trouble breathing. What is this condition?

Respiratory syncytial virus (RSV) strikes many babies in the first two years of life (especially in winter and spring), although it usually results in nothing more than a cold. Obviously your nephew is one of the exceptions who developed bronchiolitis, which as I've said, involves inflammation of small airways. The baby may have a runny nose, cough, and fever. You may hear wheezing when he breathes due to the narrowing of small airways and mucus production in the airways from inflammation. Some babies are hospitalized if they need extra oxygen or if they have trouble feeding because they have to work so hard to breathe. Because RSV is viral, antibiotics don't work, and we can only treat symptoms. Although RSV is the most common cause of bronchiolitis, other viruses can produce similar symptoms.

How should I treat a cough without fever?

There is no good medication for babies under a year with a cough. If the cough is from a post-nasal drip, it's helpful to clear the nasal passage with a bulb syringe. You can also try positioning the baby to be more upright.

What is croup and how is it different from a cough?

Young children from six months to three years of age are most at risk for croup, which is an infection of the upper airway usually in the area of the trachea and larynx (vocal cords). Croup can cause a harsh cough called stridor that sounds like the bark of a seal. The cough may come on suddenly, often in the middle of the night. The sound is due to narrowing and inflammation of the upper airway, usually caused by a viral infection.

To try to reduce inflammation, you can take the baby outdoors if the night air is cool and damp. Some babies receive inhalation treatments with the drug epinephrine to open up the airway, as well. However, if the baby has trouble breathing, take her to the emergency room. Steroids may be given to reduce inflammation. Croup may follow onset of a cold and has a seasonal aspect, usually appearing in fall, winter, or spring.

Perils of Parenthood

There's a honeymoon period between your childhood and having children of your own where you're very rarely sick. But viruses and other ills that affect babies can knock *you* out. Most common are those awful head colds, followed by stomach flu. They're bad enough, but at the same time you're suffering, you also have to take care of your sick baby. It can be a nightmare.

Since most baby illnesses are viruses, there's nothing much you can do to treat yourself. The same rules for your child apply to you. You may want to go to the doctor for antibiotics so you can get better, but most of the time it's a virus you've caught and antibiotics don't work. However, if a viral illness goes on longer than it should, do see a doctor. If the baby could have strep throat, you should definitely get a throat culture.

Many times, one parent escapes the bug, having already had it in the past and built up immunity. But you can get a new virus or a mutation of a virus. Fortunately, both parents rarely get sick at the same time, so you can take turns. The healthy one takes care of the baby. If you do catch the same thing, hopefully your spouse is feeling better by then.

EAR INFECTIONS

How do I know if my baby has an ear infection?

If your baby has an ear infection, she may be irritable, pull at her ear, or cry in pain when she lies down (due to increased pressure in the ear when in that position). An ear infection usually develops in the context of a cold. Fever after a few days of a cold can be a signal, as well.

There are anatomic reasons why ear infections generally follow upper respiratory infections. A baby's Eustachian tube, which connects the middle ear to the back of the nose and throat, is very small and narrow and tends to be horizontal. When babies catch a cold, the area around the tube becomes inflamed, sometimes blocking the tube itself. This causes negative pressure to build in the middle ear cavity and tends to draw fluid from surrounding tissue. Fluid is always a medium for viruses and bacteria.

Middle ear infection is known as acute otitis media (AOM). Following the infection, some children may not hear properly for four to six weeks due to persistent fluid in the middle ear cavity. Older children have a wider and more vertical Eustachian tube, which is why they tend to get fewer ear infections than babies.

Must my baby's ear infection be treated with an antibiotic?

Resistance to antibiotics is a worldwide problem that has triggered a sea change in thinking about use of these drugs. It can be hard to tell the difference between fluid in the middle ear—which may not be infected—and a bacterial middle ear infection. A baby who has fever and pain plus signs of middle ear infection is treated with antibiotics. Without fever and pain, watchful waiting may be the course of action. This is another scenario where doctors use clinical guidelines coupled with good clinical judgment. It has been demonstrated that ear infection pain can be treated adequately with painkillers such as acetaminophen. Some doctors use topical anesthetics with lidocaine to numb the tympanic membrane that lines the middle ear.

Often parents of children who have had many ear infections are tempted to buy an otoscope—an instrument that allows you to look at the eardrum—to diagnose an infection on their own and save a trip to the doctor. This is not recommended because diagnosing otitis media is more complicated than just finding a red, inflamed eardrum.

Does antibiotic treatment have other drawbacks?

All drugs have side effects. The most common side effects for antibiotics are rashes, diarrhea, and vomiting.

My child has had lots of ear infections. Should he get ear tubes?

Years ago, ear tubes (also known as myringotomy tubes) were used all the time for babies who had frequent ear infections. These are small ventilation tubes that are placed by an ear, nose, and throat specialist to keep the middle ear cavity open. The tubes may allow fluid to drain out. Ear tubes are rarely used today, due to concerns about using general anesthesia, possible complications, and other issues.

What is a perforated eardrum?

Occasionally a buildup of pressure causes the eardrum to rupture or open. This is usually due to a middle ear infection and is not as serious as it sounds. There may be some temporary loss of hearing. The perforations usually heal afterward and should be checked by a physician.

What could happen if an ear infection isn't treated?

Complications of untreated ear infections, such as mastoiditis (an infection of the bone behind the ear) and meningitis, were once serious concerns. The success of immunizations has reduced these fears, but an untreated bacterial infection can spread to other parts of the body. Although we try to restrain use of antibiotics, there are times when treatment is the prudent course. Studies are being done all the time to determine when we need to use antibiotics and for how long.

What should I do if my baby spits out the medicine?
If she refuses medicine, try distracting her and then sneaking it into her mouth. You can also try holding her nose, which opens her mouth and makes her swallow. Some parents try to mix in medication with food or drink. The risk is it's hard to know how much medication has been taken if some food is left over and isn't eaten. You can also ruin a baby's favorite dish once it has been tainted by a medicinal taste she dislikes.

OTHER COMMON CONCERNS

I've read about MRSA infections in babies. What are they?

MRSA stands for methicillin-resistant Staphylococcus aureus. Staph bacteria come in many different forms and can be present on healthy skin. However, Staph aureus can cause severe infection in many organs. In the last few years, we've seen a rise in Staph aureus infections that are resistant to the usual treatments, such as methicillin.

We're hearing more about MRSA today because of the growth of antibiotic resistance throughout the world. The incidence of MRSA has increased in babies, and MRSA may be suspected if an infant has a rash that looks like little pustules. The infection usually starts in the diaper, spreads elsewhere, and requires medical attention. A culture will be taken to confirm the diagnosis.

Can teething cause illness?

Teething, which usually begins around four to six months, is often blamed for fever, diarrhea, and a host of other maladies that have nothing to do with teething. Many times a baby is sick and people will say, "He's been teething." But for many babies, teething really doesn't cause anything except drooling and fingers in the mouth. If your baby also seems very cranky, check his gums for redness and swelling. To ease discomfort, try a teething ring containing freezable liquid. You can keep the ring in the freezer. The cold helps reduce gum inflammation.

Teething babies tend to receive too much medication. Rarely is acetaminophen necessary. Remember, babies can fuss for a host of reasons. Sometimes they are just in a bad mood.

What are the signs of dehydration in babies, and why is it so dangerous?

If you know your baby is losing fluid through diarrhea, frequent urination, vomiting, or fever, watch for symptoms of dehydration like crying with no tears, a dry mouth without saliva, droopiness or irritability. If she has not voided for eight hours or more, she could be dehydrated. Diapers today are quite absorbent, and it can be hard to detect urine. If in doubt, the baby should be seen by the doctor because dehydration can be fatal in small infants. Inadequate fluid intake can also cause dehydration.

What should I do if my baby has a stomach virus?

Babies can vomit and have diarrhea for all sorts of reasons, including viral gastroenteritis (otherwise known as the "stomach bug"). Be sure to discuss such symptoms with the doctor, who may want to see the baby. Instead of treating with medications, the focus may be on hydrating the baby until the virus passes. Your doctor may tell you to continue to breastfeed, but also to offer an electrolyte solution such as Pedialyte to replace essential electrolytes that may have been lost. If the baby won't take the breast or a bottle, you can use a dropper or syringe (minus the needle) to drip fluid into his mouth.

My friend's baby has a urinary tract infection. How will I know if my baby develops one?

Urinary tract infections are very difficult to diagnose because babies can't tell you if they have pain when they urinate and you may not notice that they're peeing more frequently than usual. Fever is the main way to detect a UTI, although babies get fever for all sorts of reasons. Sometimes you can detect an odor to the urine when there's an infection, but dehydration can also make urine smell. If your baby has a temperature for more than forty-eight hours (sooner if he doesn't look right), call your pediatrician. A doctor who is concerned about the possibility of a UTI will probably do a urine test for confirmation.

Urinary tract infections are one of the most common bacterial infections. They are more common in girls than boys—except in the first six months, when UTIs turn up more frequently in boys (especially uncircumcised males).

I heard a child at our day care center has roseola. What is that?

Roseola is a viral illness caused by herpes virus 6. It commonly affects babies and toddlers. Roseola begins with several days of high temperature and irritability. The fever then breaks and goes away. A fine red rash all over the body, lasting up to two days, follows. Roseola is contagious, but difficult to diagnose until the rash develops. Reappearance of high temperature after the rash is gone signals it is probably *not* roseola. The rash does not require treatment. Manage the fever as you would any fever.

> ## Call the Doctor for These Signs and Symptoms in Your Baby
>
> Temperature of 100.4 degrees or more in a baby less than eight weeks old
>
> Persistent temperature for more than forty-eight hours in a baby over eight weeks old
>
> Fever that develops after a baby is sick for a few days
>
> Vomiting and/or diarrhea
>
> Respiratory distress
>
> Unexplained irritability or lethargy
>
> Loss of appetite
>
> No wet diapers for eight hours or more
>
> Unfamiliar rash
>
> Wheezing
>
> Unusual urine odor
>
> Blood in the stool
>
> Persistent cough

One of my baby's eyes is always teary and there's crust on it in the morning. Is something wrong?

This is most likely a blocked tear duct if the white of the eye is clear and there is just a small amount of crust. There's a small duct that leads from the corner of the eye, where the tears are produced by the lachrymal glands. Tears should travel through this lachrymal duct to the sinuses. The duct may be blocked by a small web or may be too narrow to drain properly. Because the tears cannot drain into the duct, they tend to overflow and surround the eye. Any time fluids are blocked, they are prone to infection. Usually a blocked naso-lacrimal duct produces a whitish mucusy discharge that can be cleared using a warm cotton ball or facecloth. Some doctors recommend massage of the duct to help open up the canal.

The duct tends to open after a year of age, and the blockage clears up by itself. If not, a surgical procedure is performed under anesthesia to dilate the duct with a probe.

There is also an outside chance the teary eyes and crust are symptoms of conjunctivitis, an inflammation of the tissue lining of the eyeball and the insides of the lids. The whites of the eyes are red if it's conjunctivitis, which can be bacterial or viral. Conjunctivitis is a contagious condition that an infant would probably have caught from an older sibling. Pus or colored drainage from the eye right after birth should be reported to your doctor.

What is meningitis and can it be prevented?

Meningitis is a serious infection of the spinal cord fluid that can be viral (most common) or bacterial. Most types of viral meningitis are managed with supportive care; occasionally an antiviral can be used along with fluids and pain medicine. Bacterial meningitis is treated with antibiotics, but it must be detected early or it can rapidly become fatal. The highest risk for bacterial meningitis is from six to eighteen months of age. Many strains of bacterial meningitis can be prevented with immunizations.

What are the symptoms of meningitis?

Headache, fever, irritability, stiff neck, a bulging soft spot or fontanel, lethargy, and vomiting can be signs of viral or bacterial meningitis. Petechiae, which are little red dots on the skin that don't go away when pressed, appear in bacterial meningitis, although they also appear in other situations. Due to immunization, we're seeing a lot less of meningitis. When children turn twelve we vaccinate against meningoccocal meningitis, a virulent bacterial meningitis that kills swiftly. If meningitis is suspected, a spinal tap is done and the culture is sent to a lab for confirmation.

What is strep throat and how can I recognize it?

Actually, strep is extremely rare in young babies unless a sibling has it. I rarely see this until three or four years of age, although an older child can bring it home to a baby. Symptoms include fever, refusal to eat, and fussiness (since babies can't tell you their throat is sore). If strep is suspected, a throat swab is tested or a rapid strep test is done in the office. Antibiotics are prescribed only if the diagnosis is confirmed. Most sore throats are viral and do not require antibiotics.

My baby is always getting mosquito bites and I'm afraid he'll get Eastern equine encephalitis or West Nile virus. My husband says I'm overreacting. Am I?

Both of these infections are rare, but if you're in a mosquito area it's always wise to prevent bites, if possible. Avoid being outdoors at dawn and at dusk hours, which are peak times for mosquitoes. Use mosquito netting if available, and keep the baby covered as much as possible. If the baby is getting bitten and can't be covered up, use a spray with DEET. But try to avoid bug sprays if you can.

Can babies get headaches? How do you treat if they do?

We have no way of knowing. It's fair to assume if they have a temperature they probably have a headache because headache is common with fever. You're probably going to treat the fever with acetaminophen or ibuprofen, which will relieve the headache, too.

Which rashes are signs of illness, rather than allergies?

Babies get a lot of rashes, especially if they are fair-skinned, but most have nothing to do with being sick. A rash can, however, be a symptom of certain illnesses, such as roseola and Fifth Disease, a benign viral infection characterized by red cheeks that look like the baby has been slapped. Hand,

Foot, and Mouth disease, which is caused by a Coxsackie virus, tends to produce little blisters in the back of the mouth, palms of hands, balls of the feet, and occasionally on the buttocks.

Babies can also get yeast infections and bacterial rashes on the skin, such as staph or strep. Staph or strep rashes appear as pustules, especially in the diaper area, and usually are treated with oral antibiotics or sometimes a topical antibiotic cream.

My pediatrician said he noticed a heart murmur at the last checkup, but it was an innocent heart murmur. What does that mean?

An "innocent heart murmur" is not a sign of disease. Instead, the term refers to a sound produced by blood flowing across a heart valve—a common and normal physiologic sound of no consequence. There's no reason for concern. If a baby with a heart murmur has blue lips, shortness of breath, or just doesn't look well, call the doctor immediately. There could be something structurally wrong with the heart, and the baby may need a referral to a pediatric cardiologist for an evaluation and echocardiogram. Most serious heart disease is picked up before birth or right afterward.

Some heart murmurs are caused by small holes in the heart that usually disappear as the baby gets older. Your doctor will tell you whether the murmur should be checked regularly.

When is the baby sick enough to keep home from day care?

If your baby has a fever, is vomiting, has diarrhea, or an eye discharge, it is better to keep him home. Although it may be tempting to send him in and hope for the best, you probably will get a call from day care as soon as you get to work anyway.

Talking Together

Day after day of well-baby visits and anxious phone calls have given me a window into the obsessions of new mothers and fathers. Sometimes the worry is unwarranted; other times, the baby really is sick, and concerted action by both of you is required. Certainly the first fever throws fear into the hearts of most parents. At such times, try to talk together about your anxieties instead of snapping at each other because you're scared the baby's "cold" is actually pneumonia. This kind of sharing gives you perspective and draws you closer. Parents often have different reactions to illness in their children, based on their own wiring and personal health scares. Some people become germ-phobic and super protective of their baby; others may be more relaxed, and some would say "cavalier" in their view of illness and germs. Try not to overreact to the logistics of managing illness (especially if the baby is in day care) and avoid the blame game.

Also discuss and decide in advance issues such as "Who will take the sick baby to the doctor?" In some families, it's dad. Who will leave work to pick up if day care calls that the baby is sick and must go home? Talk about alternative arrangements if the baby gets sick while one of you is out of town or in a meeting.

SICK BABIES, HEALTHY BABIES

Babies are resilient. They get sick quickly and they get well quickly. Of course it's important to do your best to keep your baby healthy and strong. But you can count on several illnesses during the first year unless he has no contact at all with other children. The fact is, each time your baby is sick, he is building antibodies. By school age he should be more resistant to many infections. It is part of childhood to be sick at times, just as caring for a sick baby is also part of parenting.

CHAPTER 11

Injuries and Accidents— Call the Medics

This chapter covers:

- Falls and head injuries
- Choking and swallowing objects
- Poison, burns, and drowning
- Other injuries and accidents

Every parent's nightmare is an "Oops, I just dropped the baby" moment. The fact is you're likely to experience this and/or other mishaps at one time or another in the first year—no matter how careful and watchful you are. Accidents can (and do) happen as your baby grows and moves around in the world, and because *you're* only human. That doesn't mean you stop your baby from exploring his world. Despite potential hazards everywhere, you do have to allow exploration for healthy development.

These are the questions new parents tend to ask me about handling injuries and using appropriate safety measures. The answers will help you to prevent accidents, and take effective action when necessary.

FALLS

What if I *do* drop the baby? How badly can she be hurt?
Fortunately nature has fashioned babies' skulls to withstand such accidents. In all my years of practice I've rarely seen a baby seriously hurt by an unintentional drop. It usually takes a direct, severe blow to the head to do damage. On the other hand, do be vigilant about slipping or tripping while holding the baby. Watch out for toys lying on the floor; remove loose

scatter rugs; and hold on to the railing when using stairs. Try not to multitask when carrying the baby—and that includes talking on the cell phone. You can also always go back and get that cup of caffeine after securing the baby.

Is it okay to leave my baby alone for a minute on the changing table?

Never leave the baby alone on an elevated structure. Some babies roll over very early or can maneuver their way off changing tables (and sofas) before they can roll over. Do your best to minimize falls. I urge parents to keep at least one hand on the child at all times, right from the beginning. Why take a chance?

My mother says it's dangerous to put the baby in an infant seat on the kitchen counter. Do you agree?

Yes, I do agree. I've seen babies push the whole seat off the counter with them in it. Some hyperactive, colicky, or angry babies can arch their backs and flip over. Falls abound when parents don't realize that the baby is ready to move around, which can even occur right after birth. Although it's easier on adults (and their backs) to place the baby up high (and away from curious family pets), it is not a safe practice.

How do I know if a fall is serious?

Falls are the leading cause of non-fatal unintentional injuries in children. It's usually traumatic to the family when a fall happens. But try not to panic. Take a step back and look at where and how the baby landed. A fall of several feet from a changing table to a hard wood floor can do damage. You need to evaluate the situation. Did he cry right away? Many babies take a pause and even hold their breath after a fall that has frightened them. The breath holding may last for several seconds and can be very frightening to witness. All you can do is wait until breathing resumes.

Next, check for any bumps, cuts, or bruises, and see if he can move his arms and legs. If so, you can pick him up and console him. The best remedy for a lump on the head or elsewhere is ice applied to the area. Place ice cubes in a plastic bag and wrap the bag in a towel. (Do not put the ice directly on the baby's skin.) You can also buy prepackaged cold packs at the drug store that you can keep in the freezer ready for use.

Damaged blood vessels in the second layer of skin may start bleeding if the baby hit his head hard in the fall. Blood and fluid pour into the tissue, causing a goose egg. Apply ice immediately to stop the bleeding and prevent accumulation of fluid, which appears as a swelling. Expect loud protests because babies don't like ice. Try distracting him with a video or a toy in order to keep the ice pack in place at least for a few minutes.

Once you've applied ice, get a sense of whether he is alert, calming down, and getting back to normal. Look at his pupils, which should be the same size in both eyes. If one pupil is larger than the other (assuming they've been equal in size in the past) that can be a sign of head injury. If the baby doesn't seem to be himself in any significant way, go to the emergency room. If you are not sure about this or any other injury, call your baby's doctor. In a typical afternoon, I see about twenty children and maybe six are there for checkups. The rest are sick or injured babies who come in the same day.

Often you'll feel guilty and responsible when these things happen, but don't let emotions get in the way of looking at the child objectively. If he is gurgling and happy and there are no obvious signs of injury, just relax. Overreacting will frighten the baby, who will sense that you are upset. It's perfectly okay to nurse if he wants to feed, or offer a bottle or pacifier.

What should I do if the baby turns blue and passes out?

It's rare that a baby loses consciousness after a fall, but if she does, she needs immediate evaluation at the emergency room. Sometimes babies have what is called altered consciousness, which means she may be hard to arouse or extremely irritable. This warrants a trip to the emergency room, too.

Why are head injuries so worrisome?

Head injuries in babies that result in large bumps or hematomas on the skull, altered consciousness or loss of consciousness, or repeated vomiting or unexpected behavioral changes may indicate skull fracture or bleeding within or on top of the brain. Such bleeding causes pressure within a fixed space (the skull) that leads to brain injury. A neurosurgeon can evacuate the blood if it is around the brain to prevent permanent damage.

I heard that it's dangerous to allow a child to go to sleep after a head injury. Is that true?

In years past, we recommended waking the baby every few hours after a fall to be sure he wasn't unconscious. Arousal checks after a head injury have recently been re-evaluated because there is no data to support these wake-up drills. But be sure to get your doctor's okay to let the baby sleep.

What if the baby hurt her leg or arm?

Occasionally we see fractures in arms or legs after an infant's fall. If the baby isn't moving a limb after a fall or seems unusually fussy when moving, wrap the arm or leg with a blanket and go to the doctor.

Children, including babies, have a very vulnerable area at the end of their bones where growth occurs, called a growth plate. Growth plate fractures are not usually serious, but they must be identified and immobilized for a period of healing.

How do I know if an injury is a fracture or a sprain?

Fracture involves damage to the bone and appears as a crack or wrinkle on an X-ray. A sprain, on the other hand, is a soft tissue injury—usually to a ligament or tendon, which attaches muscle to bone or bone to bone. A fracture is more serious because it needs to be immobilized (usually with a cast) for optimal healing. Babies under a year rarely get sprains. They do get bruises, which are basically bleeding in the second layer of skin causing discoloration.

My baby, who is just beginning to walk, keeps falling and hitting his head. How can I prevent this?

The main thing to do is try to babyproof the environment. Toddlers "toddle" and they hit things. By the end of the first year, they impulsively lunge for objects. Some people remove everything from a room where the baby will play. Sharp edges on furniture must be padded. It's important to let babies move around and investigate their surroundings, but they don't need to climb on the coffee table. In a setting that's not your own home (and isn't babyproofed), try to be extra alert to dangers.

When my friend's baby fell, his tooth went through his lip. There was blood everywhere. What should I do in such a situation?

The most important action for bleeding is to locate the source and put pressure with clean gauze directly on the affected area (if possible). Hold the pressure for five minutes to allow clotting to occur. Gauze is preferable to tissue because the latter tends to stick to the wound. There is a tendency to panic at the sight of heavy bleeding. Instead, try to stay calm and immobilize the child. Put him in your lap, and hold his arms and legs down if you're alone and have no help. Once bleeding has stopped, put an ice pack on the area to prevent swelling. Although such injuries are dramatic, they usually heal quickly. Occasionally a stitch may be needed on the lip if there is a large laceration that continues to bleed.

My twelve-month-old baby, who was walking fine, now refuses to walk. What could be the reason?

It's very important that your pediatrician see her because the problem could be something serious like a fracture or a joint infection. On the other hand, it might be minor. Questions to ask yourself include: Does she have a fever, which suggests infection? Is there a history of injury to her foot or leg? Do her shoes fit properly? Babies are superior to adults in knowing when to avoid painful activity. If a part of the body hurts, they will refuse to use or put weight on it. There is also a condition called toxic synovitis, an inflammation of the joint that can occur without any apparent reason. The discomfort from this benign condition may temporarily stop a child from walking.

My friend wants to give me a baby walker her child has outgrown. I've heard that walkers are dangerous. Is that so?

Yes. Baby walkers with wheels have caused injuries to thousands of babies a year, mainly due to tumbles down stairs or falls from the walker itself. Almost one in ten injuries from a walker involves skull fracture. The AAP wants to prohibit the manufacture and sale of walkers in the United States. Canada has banned the sale of new and used walkers since 2004. Ironically, mobile walkers do not facilitate early walking and even delay motor skill development.

Prevent Falls

- Don't leave your baby alone on a sofa, changing table, or bed.
- Use safety gates at the top and bottom of stairs.
- Don't sit your baby in a baby carrier or car seat on a counter.
- Do not use a baby walker with wheels.
- Always use safety straps on high chairs, strollers, and baby swings.
- Be alert to slippery floors from splashes or spills in the bathroom or kitchen, and tape down the ends of scatter rugs (or remove them altogether).

CHOKING AND SWALLOWING OBJECTS

The entire pacifier got caught in my nephew's mouth. What should you do in that situation?

He must have a very wide mouth. In a case like this, you want to get a lever of some sort, such as a toothbrush, that you can slide into the mouth and behind the pacifier to pop it out. You don't have to worry that the pacifier will pass down the esophagus. The pacifier is too big.

Should I learn the Heimlich maneuver in case my baby chokes?

Yes, if it's at all possible. Fast action can save your baby's life, but don't wait for an emergency. Learn now how to do the Heimlich maneuver for babies, which is different from what you'd do for an older child or an adult. The Red Cross offers courses in the maneuver (and in CPR) throughout the country. It's a good idea to take one *before* anything happens. For a course locale near you, check out the Red Cross Web site at www.redcross.org.

There may be other courses available in your community, too. Ask your pediatrician if she knows of any. You can also practice instructions offered online, such as on www.webmd.com, but check out your form with the doctor to make sure you're doing it correctly. You don't want to cause any harm to the child. You have some time to develop expertise because choking is unlikely to be an issue until the baby is around four or five months old, and eating solid foods and putting objects in her mouth.

It's also a good idea to find out if there's someone nearby who can help in a crisis. A nurse or a fireman who knows the Heimlich and CPR is an ideal neighbor to have.

What do I do if my baby chokes on something like a piece of toast?

First, give him a chance to clear it himself because the natural cough reflex should work. If he keeps coughing, get up from your chair and get ready to interact if you have to.

Unless you can clearly see the food or foreign body and can easily dislodge it (rarely the case), do not try to do a finger sweep, as you may push the object farther down the trachea or breathing tube and make the situation worse. If the baby stops breathing, call 911, and do the Heimlich for babies if you know it—or scream for that neighbor.

My ten-month-old niece swallowed a nickel. What should I do if something like that happens to my baby?

Incidents of babies swallowing bizarre foreign objects do happen, as any emergency room doctor will attest. Beware of marbles, grapes, and coins. The danger with most coins occurs when they are first swallowed because a baby can choke on them. A coin that makes it past the larynx into the esophagus and goes down usually is excreted without any problem. Check every stool to make sure it passes. However,

> ### Exorcising Guilt
>
> Every parent (and I do mean *every*) feels tremendous guilt for causing unintentional injury to the baby, or failing to prevent it. But we all make mistakes, no matter how much we love our children—and some incidents are simply unavoidable. Once babies are mobile, they can get into anything. It's difficult to stay ahead of them. Be kind to yourself and ask these questions:
>
> - Was I fully present with my child or was I multitasking on the phone, the BlackBerry, or cooking? You can't be as alert to potential hazards when your attention is divided.
> - Was I impaired, intoxicated, medicated, or distracted when the event occurred?
> - Did I anticipate the possibility of this accident?
> - What other accidents are waiting to happen?
> - What can I do now to prevent other accidents?
>
> See Chapter 8 for ways to childproof your home. Review your childproofing list periodically in case it needs updating to reflect the baby's new or anticipated developmental abilities. And let go of your guilt. What's important is learning from mistakes and experience.

if the baby seems uncomfortable, an X-ray may be necessary to find the coin's location.

What are the most dangerous foreign bodies babies may swallow?

The foreign bodies we worry about most have sharp edges, such as parts of toys that can get stuck or cause damage on the way down the digestive tract. Items that contain corrosive chemicals can be harmful if they do not pass out through the stool. The doctor will try to locate the object via X-ray or may elect to remove a harmful object under anesthesia with an endoscope (a long fiber-optic tube with a light). Most objects pass right through the GI (gastrointestinal) tract.

Recently a baby I saw had swallowed a small round cell phone battery. An X-ray of the stomach found it, and the father watched for it in the stool. When it did not show up, another X-ray followed several days later and the battery was not seen. Although the father had not found the battery in the stool, it was assumed to have safely passed because the child was fine.

Be alert to parts of broken toys that can be swallowed. The best idea is to throw out broken toys. Latex balloons don't belong in the house because babies can swallow pieces of them. And pay attention to recommended age guidelines on toy packaging. An appropriate toy for an older child may be dangerous for a baby.

POISON

What should I do if my child swallows a poisonous substance?

Once babies are scooting around the house, they can get into chemicals or cleaning supplies under the sink in the bathroom or kitchen. Visitors' purses are another attractive nuisance. Babies find the contents fascinating and can grab pills or other medications and put them in their mouths. Child-resistant caps make it harder to open pill containers, but the caps are not foolproof. Anything that falls on the rug is fair game, too. Babies get into trouble when adults are chatting and distracted.

If the baby eats the deodorant or the nail polish remover or other possibly harmful substances, first call the National

Poison Control hotline at 1-800-222-1222 immediately for advice on what to do. (Keep that number posted prominently near the phone.) Children five and under are involved in half the calls. Depending on what has happened, you may be told to go to the emergency room, where charcoal may be given to bind to the poisonous substance. Charcoal helps prevent the chemical from being absorbed. A baby that ingests cardiac medication from grandma's purse may have to be monitored with a respiratory or cardiac monitor.

I heard that ipecac is no longer used when a child ingests poison. Why?

Ipecac was long recommended to induce vomiting in children who might have eaten poisonous substances. But there's been a change in thinking about ipecac. We now know it causes repeated vomiting that can lead to aspiration. We don't want a child to vomit and risk bringing up toxic material through the esophagus or throat.

What if I'm not sure whether the baby ate poison or not?

It's best to call Poison Control regardless. Sometimes you can tell by the color or the residue on the tongue or a smell in the baby's mouth, but it may be hard to be certain.

BURNS

How should I deal with burns?

Babies manage to get around whether they're walking yet or not. If there's a hot stove, hot plate, or hot iron around, little hands can find it. You'll know about it because the baby will start screaming in pain. The best thing to do is immediately run cold water over the affected area to prevent any further burning of tissue. (Even if the baby's hand is removed from the source of the burn, there can be continued tissue damage.) Cold water also flushes away fluid, such as hot tea, involved with the burn.

The Three Types of Burns

First-degree burn. This category of burn is superficial and affects only the outer layer of skin. The area is red and painful.

Second-degree burn. This is more serious, penetrates to the second layer of skin, and involves blistering. Do not pop the blisters because the wall of the blister protects against infection.

Third-degree burn. This is the most damaging burn. It destroys the first and second layer of skin, as well as some nerve endings, which is why this type of burn can be painless.

Treat a first-degree burn by running cold water over it. Gently dry the area and apply a cold pack. A second- or third-degree burn must be seen by a physician, who will probably dress it with an antibiotic burn cream called Silvadene cream (silver sulfadiazine) or another topical antibiotic cream. There are special wraps that won't stick that you can use for burns.

What is a safe hot water temperature to avoid scalding?

Set the water heater temperature in your home at 120 degrees or less, and always test the baby's bath water with your hand to make sure it isn't hotter than you thought. Of course scalding can also occur in other scenarios. Never drink hot tea or coffee while holding the baby. It's just too easy for spills to happen. Turn handles on pots toward the back of the stove to prevent roving hands from grabbing them.

What other precautions should I take?

Do you know how to use a fire extinguisher? It won't do you any good hanging on the wall if you don't know what to do with it. Install one or more smoke alarms on each floor. Make sure matches and cigarette lighters are out of reach or locked away. Cover electrical outlets with caps to prevent your baby from sticking his finger into the socket. Be aware that babies can pull on the loose hanging cord of a hot iron or lamp.

DROWNING

I don't have a pool. Do I still have to worry about my baby drowning?

According to research funded by the National Institute of Child Health and Human Development (NICHD), most infants drown at home—primarily in the bathtub. Toddlers are more likely to drown in a pool.

What preventive measures should I take?

Never leave the baby alone in the bathtub, even for a second, or near a pool. Keep the toilet seat cover down, and don't leave a pail of water around. Babies can drown in an inch or two of water. As I was writing this book, an eleven-month-old drowned in a mop bucket in New York City. If you have a hot tub, cover it for safety.

MISCELLANEOUS INJURIES

How can I prevent suffocation or strangulation?

A 2009 study found that U.S. infant mortality rates from accidental smothering or strangulation in beds, cribs, or couches quadrupled between 1984 and 2004. Precautions you can take include putting the baby to sleep on her back, choosing a safe crib (one with slats no more than $2\frac{3}{8}''$ apart), and excluding soft bedding like quilts and pillows from the crib. Note that babies can strangle by getting entangled with window blind cords.

I accidentally scratched my baby's eye. The eye is tearing and he's been crying. What should I do?

It's possible you caused a small corneal abrasion. The cornea is a thin tissue over the eyeball and is easy to scratch, causing redness, tearing, and pain. Scratches usually heal within forty-eight hours. This injury should be checked by your physician, who can put a dye in the eye and then highlight a scratch on the cornea, if there is one, with a special light called a Wood's Lamp. Some doctors prescribe antibiotic ointment to prevent infection. The eye used to be patched to prevent the lid from fluttering back and forth, but that is no longer recommended.

I slammed the baby's finger in the door. What should I do?

This happened to me. I didn't realize that my grandson had his fingers in the hinge of a door when I closed it. I felt so terrible that I hadn't noticed his hand. The first thing to do is ice the finger or hand if you can to minimize swelling. Some parents say, "Well we tried to but he wouldn't let us." This is one situation where you have to sit the child in your lap, hold him down, and get that ice pack on. If there is significant swelling, call your doctor. The finger will probably have to be X-rayed. You may think a finger looks fine, but little bones are vulnerable to fractures in the growth plate area. Fractures heal quickly and do well, yet they do need to be seen. My grandson didn't need an X-ray because his finger wasn't swollen or discolored and he could move all his fingers.

My baby bumped her nose, which is bleeding. What should I do?

Nose bleeds are very common because blood vessels in the lining of the nose are very fragile and close to the surface and bleed easily. Pinch the nostrils together and help the baby sit slightly forward for five minutes until clotting occurs. Try not to rub or touch the nose for a few hours afterward. Nose bleeds may also occur when the baby has a winter cold, and the nasal mucosa is dried by heat in your home. After you've stopped the bleeding, dip a cotton swab in some petroleum jelly and apply to the inside of the nostril. A humidifier in the baby's room can be helpful, or put a pan of water in the room. Just remember to change the water daily to prevent growth of fungus.

My baby walked barefoot on the deck and got lots of little splinters in his feet. What's the best way to handle this?

This is a reminder of the role of shoes for walking babies—to keep their feet warm and to protect the feet from foreign bodies. Most of the time, the splinters are embedded in the upper layer of skin. They will take care of themselves, don't cause any problems, and don't need to be removed. But if splinters penetrate the second layer of skin, where there are nerve endings and blood, splinters can be painful and may get infected. They must be removed. If you have sharp forceps at home and someone to hold the baby, you can remove these splinters. If not, the pediatrician should do it. It's very hard to get out a deep splinter when the baby is screaming and kicking. The old method of burning a sewing needle in a flame to sterilize it isn't very efficient.

How can I keep my baby safe in the car?

Your local police can help you install a baby car seat properly. Be sure to use the safety straps even if you're just driving a

> ## *Talking Together*
>
> Nothing beats preparation for emergency situations. Discuss in advance "What will we do if…?" What *will* you do if the nurse next door is not home? Know the location of the nearest emergency room and how to get there. If you would ordinarily go to another hospital, the baby can be stabilized at the nearest place and can always be switched to your preferred hospital later. Anticipating emergencies and practicing what to do will increase your confidence and help you work together. Consider taking a Red Cross course as a couple. Topics covered are usually CPR, choking, bleeding, etc. I used to teach a course in my practice, and it was usually sold out.
>
> Is one of you overprotective (or unrealistic about real dangers)? This is another issue to talk about. Share your feelings and fears. Were you (or your spouse) brought up in a fearful household? There's a line between sensible caution and inhibiting your child from the exploration needed for healthy development. If you and your spouse can't come to agreement, consider talking together with your pediatrician, who can bring knowledge and perspective to differences over what's safe and what's excessive restriction.

block or two. Babies should sit in rear-facing car seats until they weigh at least twenty pounds and are one year of age.

READY FOR ANYTHING?

Babies under a year of age have the highest child mortality rate from accidents. Never underestimate your child and always try to stay ahead of him. When there's a baby in the house, anything can happen. Lumps, bumps, scrapes, and myriad misadventures are inevitable as children master rolling over, crawling, standing, walking, and grabbing. You can, however, take precautions and know what to do when minor (or major) emergencies occur. There are risks in life, especially as babies turn into toddlers. Fortunately, many accidents are preventable, and babies are a lot tougher than you think.

Bear in mind, too, that some accidents can occur due to problems in baby equipment. Even after a product is approved, the item can be recalled later for safety concerns. Be alert to announcements of recalls in the media.

CHAPTER 12

Allergies—
What You Need to Know

This chapter covers:
- Facts about allergies
- Food allergies
- Handling allergic reactions
- Asthma, eczema, and other allergies

It happens often. Panicked parents arrive at my office with a baby covered with a red rash. Her face is puffed into a moon shape. Or the baby has itchy red welts all over his body. In both cases, the problem is an allergy. Because allergies are common and the field of allergies and immunology is constantly changing, you may hear conflicting information about these conditions. Yet there is no doubt that eczema, asthma, and peanut allergies are on the rise in babies.

The questions and answers that follow will help clear up any understandable confusion about what is and isn't an allergy and how to proceed when an allergy is diagnosed.

ALLERGY EDUCATION

What *are* allergies?

Allergic reactions involve the immune system. The body may react to a certain food or environmental trigger by producing a rash, wheezing, or swelling. The substance in question, called an allergen, causes a release of chemicals. The result is an allergic reaction, which can occur on the skin in the form of a rash, or in the eyes, nose, throat, lungs, or digestive system. The allergic response occurs any time the person is exposed to the allergen and may intensify with each exposure.

What are common signs of allergies in babies?

Hives (big red itchy welts that can appear anywhere on the body) are the most typical allergic rash. But sometimes facial swelling, vomiting, constipation, irritability, or diarrhea can signal an allergic reaction. Blood and mucus in the stool are common in babies allergic to cow's milk protein. Respiratory distress may occur in a severe reaction. Bear in mind, however, that sometimes allergies are misdiagnosed. It is important that a doctor confirm that the reaction is really an allergy.

Why do babies get allergies?

Allergies are usually acquired over time, and there is usually a genetic link. If eczema, asthma, or food allergies run in the family, your baby may be susceptible.

How are allergies diagnosed in a baby?

Often allergies are diagnosed by history alone, i.e., your baby eats a strawberry and develops hives right afterward. The pediatrician may refer you to an allergist, who can perform a skin test and blood tests. The skin or "prick" test uses tiny needles with small amounts of the offending allergen to see if a local reaction occurs. This is thought to be the most reliable test. RAST testing and IGE testing are blood tests that measure antibody levels against the allergen and are thought to be slightly less reliable than the skin test.

FOOD ALLERGIES

What are the most common food allergies?

Food allergies occur when specific foods or food additives are ingested. Eight types of food account for over 90 percent of allergic reactions: milk, eggs, peanuts, tree nuts (such as almonds), fish, shellfish, soy, and wheat.

What are the most common food allergies in babies?

Allergies to strawberries, peanut butter, citrus, tomatoes, and food coloring are common. A reaction can even be fatal. There are about 9,500 hospitalizations of children annually related to food allergies.

Babies allergic to the protein in cow's milk, which is present in both formula and breast milk (due to dairy in the mother's diet) may be switched to soy formulas that are made from soybeans and are lactose-free. However, some babies are also allergic to soy and may have to be switched to an elemental formula (which does not contain cow's milk protein or soy-based protein). For more information on cow's milk protein allergy, see Chapter 2.

Is lactose intolerance the same as an allergy to milk?

Lactose intolerance isn't an allergy. Instead it's the loss (usually partial) of a lactose enzyme in the small intestines that breaks down lactose sugar. There are two types of lactose intolerance. Primary lactose intolerance involves an inability to break down lactose sugars from birth and is extremely rare. Secondary lactose intolerance is an acquired condition where the baby temporarily loses the ability to digest lactose sugar. This condition usually occurs after long bouts of diarrhea and clears up when the baby is put on a lactose-free formula for a short time. Parents often confuse lactose intolerance with an allergy to cow's milk protein and change the baby's formula unnecessarily. Even some doctors are confused about the diagnosis.

How has the thinking about preventing or minimizing food allergies changed?

Theories about food allergies in babies abound. At one time, infants were exposed to all sorts of foods early on, including eggs, whole milk, or whatever the parents were eating.

Later it was believed that certain foods should be withheld from babies until six months of age or even later to avoid allergies.

Current thinking falls somewhere in between. If your baby shows signs of being allergy-prone, foods such as egg whites, dairy, nut products, wheat, fish, and certain fruits are withheld until the child is older. For babies without any sign of allergic tendencies, solid foods are now introduced between four to six months, with certain nut products and dairy introduced later.

Why have food allergies increased?

Food allergies have increased in the United States and in other parts of the world for unknown reasons. Roughly twelve million Americans suffer from them. According to the CDC, one in four children under the age of eighteen, and one in twenty under age three has a food or digestive allergy.

Are there gender differences in susceptibility to food allergies?

The incidence of food allergies in boys and girls is roughly the same. However, there are age and ethnic differences. For example, Hispanic children are less likely to suffer food allergies than Caucasian or black children. Children under five are more likely to get food allergies than older children.

Can children outgrow food allergies?

Food allergies are more prevalent in children than adults, but the majority of youngsters will outgrow these allergies. Children are less likely to outgrow a nut allergy; parents should not reintroduce nuts to an allergic child without medical supervision.

My baby is allergic to cow's milk. Can she have yogurt or ice cream?

Most babies who have cow's milk protein allergy usually outgrow it by twelve months of age. It's prudent to wait to introduce dairy products like yogurt until a year, but only in consultation with your pediatrician.

Should I avoid offering my baby certain foods?

Your pediatrician will provide guidelines for food introduction. Usually we start with baby cereal fortified with iron and then add one new food every few days so that we will know which food is to blame if a reaction occurs. If your baby has shown signs of being allergic to a certain food, that food should be avoided until the baby is older. The food should not be reintroduced without direction from an allergist. An allergist who thinks a child may have outgrown a food allergy may test for it in the office to observe any reaction and provide treatment, if necessary.

I thought that nuts should be banned until age three, but now I read that it may not be a good idea to do that. Which is it?

Peanut allergies have increased—and unlike most food allergies, which are outgrown, this one tends to persist. Reactions to these allergies can be life threatening. The ban until age three hopes to delay exposure. However, this restriction is currently being reviewed due to recent research findings. When allergic children received tiny doses of peanuts daily, followed by gradually increased amounts, most were able to tolerate the peanuts. This is a desensitization approach.

What are the symptoms of a peanut allergy?

Reactions can vary and may include a swollen tongue, hives, wheezing, or constriction of the throat. Abdominal pain, vomiting, or diarrhea can also be signs.

How to Handle Allergic Reactions

If your baby has been diagnosed with a food allergy, always keep two medications on hand. An EpiPen Jr is an easy-to-use injectable epinephrine that is used to alleviate respiratory distress due to exposure to a known allergen. The pen is poked into the baby's thigh and the medication injected into the muscle. Your doctor will give you a few EpiPen Jrs. If your child wheezes or his tongue swells or he has any kind of respiratory distress, administer the EpiPen Jr and go to the nearest emergency room right away or call 911.

The second medication is Benadryl, an antihistamine that comes in liquid form and is given by mouth. Benadryl is used for milder reactions, such as hives. If your child has hives, administer Benadryl in a weight-based dose, and call your doctor. Watch for signs of labored breathing, excessive drooling, or color change. If you are not sure how severe the reaction is, go to the emergency room.

Is there anything else I should do to manage a peanut allergy?

Each child under sixty pounds should have at least two EpiPen Jrs. (Heavier children need the regular EpiPen, which has a larger dose of epinephrine.) Keep both Benadryl and the EpiPen Jrs on hand. These can abort an allergic reaction, but the child must also be taken to an emergency room right away. Be sure to alert day care personnel and babysitters to the allergy and what to do. A medic alert bracelet is a good idea. As soon as your child is old enough to understand, be sure he knows that he is allergic to peanut products and which foods contain peanuts. Recently certain breeds of dogs, such as Labrador retrievers have been trained to smell for peanut residue and have been life changing for children who are highly allergic to peanuts.

In an egg allergy, is the yolk or the white the problem?
Both whites and yolks can be allergens. This is an allergy babies often outgrow quickly. After a discussion with your pediatrician, you might want to test the baby to see if she tolerates eggs now. Often the child takes small tastes of baked goods made with cooked eggs to see if it still provokes a reaction. Be sure to have Benadryl on hand just in case there is a reaction.

My baby gets a rash around his mouth every time he eats sweet potatoes. Is he allergic to it?
A red rash around the mouth is called a perioral rash. If the rash is limited to that location it is probably not a true food allergy, and allergists consider it safe for the child to have that food. If there's a rash elsewhere on the body, it's a different story. A true food allergy would result in hives (big red welts) all over the body.

My baby got hives all over his body after eating fish. What should I do?
This could be a true food allergy. Until the doctor verifies it, avoid fish products. Shellfish, such as lobster, shrimp, and crab, are the most common causes of fish allergies. If your baby has a fish allergy, avoid the food and keep an EpiPen Jr and Benadryl handy at all times.

ASTHMA, ECZEMA, AND OTHER ALLERGIES

Do babies get asthma?
There is no foolproof test for asthma, especially in young children. Asthma is a diagnosis based over time using a history of the child's reaction to respiratory infections, family history,

and other allergic tendencies such as eczema or food allergies. Babies often wheeze with certain viral respiratory infections, so the asthma diagnosis may not be made until a baby is older. A tendency to wheeze with each cold may signify a possible diagnosis of asthma. Ironically, research suggests that children in day care as infants are less likely to develop asthma symptoms by age five than other youngsters.

There is a school of thought that the huge increase in asthma and allergies is due to the sterile conditions babies are exposed to today. Exposure to germs and infections in day care may build immunity. One study suggests that children who grow up on a farm and are exposed to dust and animal products are less likely to develop allergies. Another study suggested that the allergies seen in urban dwellers are often triggered by cockroach leavings.

Can I prevent my baby from getting eczema, which runs in our family?

If you live in a cold climate, keep bath time short and use a liberal amount of moisturizer after a bath and any other time you think of it. It's very important to keep a baby's skin moisturized. Areas of very dry skin can get infected if the skin breaks down. I always tell parents they cannot prevent or cure eczema. They just have to manage it until, hopefully, the child outgrows it.

Can our baby be allergic to the dog?

When babies are allergic to animal dander, it is usually obvious. They get red, itchy eyes, stuffy itchy noses, and may even wheeze after exposure. If you don't already have a pet and are thinking of a dog, research the breed if your child has allergies. Certain dogs shed less, such as Labradoodles, a cross between a Labrador and a poodle. Short-haired cats are another option. The best thing is to check with a veterinarian.

How common are skin allergies in babies?

Eczema is extremely common in infants. If your baby has cracked areas behind the knee or elbow or dry skin that progresses to scaly patches, it may be eczema. The spectrum of eczema is wide ranging from dry skin to severe broken down areas of skin. Eczema suggests an allergic tendency, which means your baby may be more prone to food allergies and/or asthma. Many babies outgrow eczema as they get older. To treat eczema, doctors may prescribe a combination of moisturizer and an anti-inflammatory, such as a topical steroid.

Do babies have respiratory allergies?

When babies wheeze, it is usually a response to an upper respiratory viral infection and may not be an allergic condition. Environmental allergens are less likely to trigger wheezing in infants.

Can babies be allergic to drugs?

Drug reactions are common. However, the rash that appears after taking amoxicillin may be a side effect, rather than an allergy to penicillin. Be sure to have your doctor look at any rash that occurs after taking a medication. If the baby has raised, itchy red welts, it may be hives, and you should stop the medication.

When should an allergy specialist see my baby?

If your baby has severe eczema that is not responding to moisturizers and low dose steroids, your doctor may refer you to a dermatologist. In cases of recurrent wheezing in the first year, referral to a pulmonologist may be appropriate. Most pediatricians are comfortable managing allergic conditions in infants and children because they are so common. Babies rarely need to see an allergist in the first year.

Do babies ever get allergy shots?

Allergy shots are given as a form of desensitization to an allergen. Small doses of an allergen are injected to stimulate a mild immune response. The hope is to eventually mute the allergic response. Babies and even young children rarely receive allergy shots.

Can babies be allergic to bee stings and airborne allergens like pollen?

They can be, but most bee sting allergies occur after an initial exposure or prior sting. Babies do tend to form large red raised marks even after a simple mosquito bite. This is a reaction to the bite but can be treated with a cold pack on the bite area. Pollen is more likely to trigger a stuffy nose or red itchy eyes, usually in older children.

Talking Together

It's important to have a conversation about each of your family medical histories because allergies do run in families. If your child has a diagnosed food allergy or is at risk for a severe reaction to any other allergy, both of you should be aware of what to do. Figure out in advance which emergency room is closest and/or best.

If you or the child's caregiver is not clear about what constitutes an allergic reaction, be sure to talk with your pediatrician. Asthma, especially, is a complicated illness and causes much confusion in families. EpiPens need to be renewed every two years and should be kept in a place that is easily accessible, such as a glove compartment in the car.

WORK WITH YOUR PEDIATRICIAN

"Early exposure to solid food is not recommended." "Waiting too long to introduce foods may deprive your baby of important nutrients." Advice about food allergies seems to change all the time. Current thinking is moving away from severe restriction of certain foods. If your baby shows no sign of allergic tendencies, and there is no family history of allergy, you can be more relaxed about the foods you introduce with the permission of your pediatrician. Although we do know the incidence of asthma has been rising, especially in economically deprived areas, the triggers for the increase are unclear.

What is clear is that allergies are everywhere. Watch for the latest news and research, and always verify a suspected allergy with the doctor to make sure it's a true allergy.

CHAPTER 13

Health Information—
Be a Savvy Consumer

This chapter covers:

- Checking whether information is valid
- The pros and cons of chat rooms, blogs, and books
- Communicating with the doctor

"Dr. McEvoy, my baby may have a sweating disorder. I've been reading online about this rare condition that causes excessive perspiration, and I think she has it." I hear such statements all the time from well-read, well-educated parents who regularly rely on the Internet for health information. In fact, 75 to 80 percent of American Internet users look for health and medical information online, according to the Pew Internet and American Life Project. The Internet is an amazingly helpful and convenient tool that puts a world of knowledge at our fingertips. Unfortunately, it can also dispense misinformation and needlessly frighten parents. In the case above, I not only had never heard of this condition, I was staring at a cute, smiling, healthy five-month-old who did not seem to have a bead of sweat on her.

Of course the Internet is not the only source of health information today. Television, radio, and print also bring us medical headlines and alerts. The media doesn't hesitate to point out the many threats to health and safety. Although the information can be useful, it sometimes serves to frighten rather than educate. The advice of well-meaning, but not always well-informed relatives can add to the confusion. Here are questions I regularly hear from parents as they deal with information overload. The answers will help you use medical information wisely and well.

NAVIGATING SOURCES

What should I do if I'm scared by information online or in the media?

From the wild west of the Internet to multiple baby care books and family members, you'll be offered all kinds of advice for your baby. But your single most important source of information is your baby's doctor. The pediatrician is building a relationship with you and your child, and has the expertise and experience necessary to assess and interpret health information.

Sometimes my mother contradicts what the pediatrician has told me. What should I do?

Vet her advice with the pediatrician because, a layman can sometimes be right on the money—and at other times totally wrong. For example, medical evidence and recommendations may have changed. A grandparent may say, "We've been putting babies to sleep on their stomachs in our family for centuries, and it's always been fine." Babies did sleep on their stomachs until the 1990s. But research has shown that sleeping on the back can help prevent SIDS. Grandparents used to think that wearing a hat prevented ear infections in babies, yet hats have nothing to do with ear infections. Sometimes family members may even insist that a home folk remedy will help colic, constipation, or other problems. But some of these concoctions can harm a baby. Why take a chance when you can easily check it out with the doctor?

What are the best Web sites for baby health information?

It's essential to separate safe and authoritative sites from those that present the opinions of people who lack credentials. There are also commercial sites whose goal is to sell products or services. The information offered may be biased.

The most reliable sites are those sponsored by government agencies such as the NIH, NICHD, CDC, FDA, the Consumer Products Safety Commission, and state or local health agencies. Other authoritative sites include those of medical centers, medical schools, universities, professional organizations such as the AAP and the AAFP, and respected organizations like La Leche League. Some prominent foundations have excellent health sites as well. See the Resources section at the back of the book for suggestions. Check whether the information is current, too. In the fast-paced world of medical research, information from just a decade ago may omit important findings since then or be outdated for other reasons. On the other hand, it may be the latest data available.

How do I know if I can believe the results of a scientific study?

It depends on who's doing the study. Is it a government study? Is the research from a medical school or university? Were the results published in journals such as *Pediatrics,* the *New England Journal of Medicine,* the *Journal of the American Medical Association, Lancet,* or other respected journals? Be a discriminating reader and discuss the research with your pediatrician, who knows what to look for, such as the number of people studied and whether there was a control group for comparison.

Autism and the MMR vaccine, cell phones and brain tumors, and microwaves and cancer are all examples of unproven, but emotional, hypotheses that have gained traction in the media. Although it may be useful to question environmental practices or medical treatments as possible suspects in causing harm, scientific studies must be done to verify theory.

Any research results should be reviewed for objectivity. Who funded the research? Did the researcher receive funds from a drug manufacturer or any other organization that may create bias when interpreting the results? Medical journals and medical schools are trying to tighten up oversight of studies, but you also should be appropriately skeptical, especially when study results seem outlandish.

MEDIA: OLD AND NEW

What is a blog and are blogs good ways to get health information?

Blogs are popular, and I have written one for www.gather .com. However, blogs can vary tremendously in the quality of content. For example, medical content for Gather health blogs was provided by Harvard Medical School faculty. Be sure the blogs you read are written and edited by a reputable source.

What do you think of parenting chat rooms online?

These can be very helpful, and there are chat rooms to suit every need, such as some for parents of premature babies or multiples. However, be wary of the validity of any advice on these sites. Remember, the contributors are other parents. You may get some great ideas from them and connect with others facing the same issues you are, but verify supposedly factual information with your doctor.

Under the auspices of Harvard Medical School, I did a live Web chat for Gather.com on disciplining children. Parents logged on from all over the country, and we had an online parenting group that was both fun and educational. Parents presented practical solutions to problems posed by other parents. I found the information from parents was accurate in some cases and way off base in others. Fortunately I was online to clarify or correct when necessary.

How about newspapers?

Respected newspapers can be excellent sources of health information because they are meticulous about getting the most recent research from reputable journals or medical schools. The caveat is they sometimes tend to select headline-grabbing research, which needs to be put in context. In one case a study suggested all smokers should have CTs of the lungs. Later it was found that what sounded like a good idea might not be. It was a valid study, but it needed critical review. It turned out CTs did not prolong life, picked up lots of false positives, and subjected people to radiation and some unnecessary procedures. In addition, the funding for the study was provided by an interested party.

Time is an important moderating influence when trying to digest breaking news on the health front. When new information comes to light, don't panic. Let other parties weigh in. With time, many "shocking revelations" may be deemed invalid. For example, remember the headlines about obesity being contagious? On the face of it, it was scary news. When the study was vetted, the results didn't tell you much that you didn't already know.

How can I evaluate TV or radio health news?

Medical news must be put into context. There are excellent professional medical journalists, such as Dr. Tim Johnson, Dr. Nancy Snyderman, or Dr. Sanjay Gupta. They select what's interesting and essential. But try to be aware of the doctor's specialty. An orthopedic surgeon may have a different perspective on a breaking story about a childhood disease than a pediatrician.

My friend's doctor sometimes gives different advice from my pediatrician. Why is this?

In pediatrics, as in most medical fields, there is usually more than one way to tackle a problem. Sometimes doctors dis-

Talking to Your Pediatrician

A relationship with your pediatrician is a two-way street. The challenge is to use the doctor as effectively as possible. Today many pediatricians have special expertise in developmental issues, sports medicine, adolescent health, or other subspecialties. In addition to offering medical advice, it's the doctor's job to explain your baby's progress and interpret information. Here's how to make the most of your pediatrician's knowledge and experience:

- Before a visit (or a phone call), write down the questions you want to ask. As you start talking back and forth, it's easy to forget something important.

- Avoid censoring yourself. No question is too silly or dumb. If it concerns you, it's essential to get answers. On the other hand, be considerate of the doctor's time and try to prioritize. If she has fit in your baby for a sick visit, stick to questions on the medical issue at hand. Some pediatric offices have a call-in time for routine telephone questions; others may welcome them at any time of the day.

- Ask your most important questions first at a well-baby checkup in case the doctor has an emergency or is behind schedule. If time is running out, ask one of the nurses or schedule another visit or phone call. You should be able to get all your questions answered in a well-child visit, but a sick visit that has been squeezed in may not be the time to ask unrelated questions.

- If you don't understand an answer or want to know more, say so. You owe it to your baby to assert yourself in this situation.

- Be friendly toward the office staff. They can often expedite your call or help in other ways. On the other hand, if a staff member is rude or not helpful, report it to the doctor. In our office, we work as a team, and if one part of the team is dysfunctional, we all suffer, including the patients.

agree. Also, every case is different. Your friend's child may not have the same medical profile as yours. Someone may tell you, "My pediatrician said my son shouldn't get the flu shot." Well if he has an egg allergy, he shouldn't. But other children should be vaccinated.

BE SELECTIVE

Which health alerts are absolutely reliable?

Alerts that come from a government agency, such as the FDA or CDC or the Consumer Products Safety Commission, or from state or local agencies are reliable. CNN, respected newspapers like the *New York Times, Wall Street Journal,* and *Washington Post* may report breaking medical news, as well.

What baby books should I buy?

If you go to the children's section of bookstores, you will see that some books are written by physicians, others by lay people. Just because a medical doctor wrote a book doesn't mean the book is authoritative. Similarly, a book written by a lay person may offer excellent information. In either case, check the experience and credentials of the author—and avoid books selling products or trendy techniques. You want real solutions to your parenting challenges, not simplistic advice or catchy titles. There are general books that are comprehensive; some are age-specific; others address certain topics such as adoptive parenting, gay parenting, parenting twins, etc. Remember, parenting is complicated. If a book promises a quick fix for a complex problem such as sleep, be wary. See the Resources section at the back of this book for some recommendations.

Talking Together

The more you know, the more confident you're going to feel. Most physicians are not threatened by well-informed parents. But handle information on the Internet and elsewhere with care. Just because you saw it online or read or heard it somewhere doesn't mean it's true. Discuss with your spouse which accurate, medically reliable Web sites you trust and will consult. Figure out how you can avoid reacting to every provocative news flash that comes across the Internet or TV screen. These are key issues to agree on.

If your child is born with a medical problem, decide together how to advocate for her in the health care system. It's important to feel your pediatrician is your ally in finding the best resources, but be prepared to do your own advocacy work. The health care system is not always user-friendly. For example, if you must see more than one specialist, ask your doctor about a good facility that offers one-stop shopping, where you can avoid getting fragmented opinions and care for your baby—and save wear and tear on yourselves. This is also a time for teamwork. One of you may be more outspoken and better at asking questions and getting clarification of information. One of you may be good at making sure all your concerns are covered. That person can assume the job whenever possible. The same approach works online if one of you is a computer whiz or an experienced researcher.

MAKING SENSE OF IT ALL

Make it a habit to critically assess reports of research or health threats by immediately asking, "What's the source? Is it authoritative and reliable?" Bring in the magazine article you want an opinion on or ask about the study you found on the Internet. Parents often educate me, and I welcome their input because they help keep me up-to-date. I'll check out what they've told me on the computer and often learn something new. Shared decision making is a priority and a good model for pediatricians. We live in the age of information and consensus-based care.

Incidentally, if you think you're overloaded now, more is on the way. For example, I've already taped three-minute videos of tips from Harvard Medical School that will appear on parents' phones.

CHAPTER 14

Work/Career—
Making Choices

This chapter covers:

- Staying home versus returning to work
- Transitioning back to work after maternity leave
- Child care options and common worries
- Productive communication with caregivers

Will one of you stay home now that the baby is here or will both of you work? Full time or part time? Now or in three years when the baby goes to nursery school? Who will watch the baby during the day? Nanny or Grandma or day care? There is no right or wrong answer—just the choice that works best for your family at this time. Whatever you decide, the reality is you're likely to feel anxiety about your choice.

The questions and answers that follow will help you focus on the considerations involved in making your decision—and how best to settle in.

CHOOSING WHAT'S BEST

We're debating who should stay home. What factors should we consider, and what's best for the baby?
There are so many considerations, beginning with "Who has a bigger paycheck?" and "Who is more career-focused and ambitious?" Other questions include: "Who wants to stay home?" "What kind of work does each of you do?" "Does one of you have to be on site at work?" If one of you can telecommute, it's a lot easier to return to work. "What is the employer's expectation?" "How family friendly is the envi-

ronment?" The answer may be "not very" if you work for a large law firm or a fast-moving venture capital or consulting firm. This should be a question dealt with by both partners, not just women.

Today I see more and more fathers who are primary caregivers. Some dads are natural nurturers and very good at it.

Do some women change their minds about returning to work after the baby arrives?

In my experience, yes. I've found it totally unpredictable which women decide to go back and which don't. Some of the most hard-driving career women opt to stay home. Often the perfectionists find they can't tolerate the stress of doing a less than good job both at work and parenting. I've seen many stay home for a time, decide to be the best mother they can be, and hope to go back later.

My husband can switch his schedule, work nights, and take care of the baby during the day when I go back to work. Is this a good idea?

This is another of those "it depends" questions. If he likes the arrangement and is good at taking care of the baby, why not? I know of one case where a couple did exactly that. He actually preferred working nights. His mother supplemented him during the day so he could get some sleep. Whatever works for you, your spouse, and the baby is a good idea. However, beware of the "ships passing in the night" syndrome where parents fulfill their role at work and at home, but their relationship flounders with reverse schedules.

I'm torn between returning to work full time or part time. Aside from finances, what are the pros and cons?

A lot has to do with what business you're in. Most women working part time wind up doing a lot of extra work for that half-time pay. It's easy to feel taken advantage of in that situation, but the trade-off can be saving your sanity. Many men and women work at home a few days a week. But of course it depends on whether your job requires face time, the attitude of your boss and colleagues, how competitive the environment is, and how much support you receive from your spouse. I find spousal support varies. In financially stressful times, part of the equality movement is that mothers are expected to pull their weight. Some fathers leave mothers on their own with child care arrangements. On the other hand, I've seen a lot of fathers stay home or work part time. The stigma of a stay-at-home father is much less than it used to be. People also transition in and out of jobs much more these days. One father stayed home for a year after he sold his company. We've come a long way from the times when the mother stayed home in suburbia and the father commuted to work.

Is it harmful to a baby when both parents work?
If both of you working gets in the way of providing a loving, stable home for your child, I would say it's a harmful arrangement. Yet by now we all know many wonderful families with two working parents. Babies need food, shelter, love, and consistency. It's an individual and personal decision how you prioritize your responsibilities to children, spouse, career, and civic duty. If you love your job or need to work, as long as you can find safe, loving, stable child care, your baby is likely to thrive.

I really want to stay home but worry I won't be a good role model for my kids if I do that. I want them see me as a complete person with many dimensions and abilities, as well as a parent and homemaker.
The best role model you can be is a thoughtful, curious person; staying home doesn't mean you can't be an inspira-

tion for your child. You're a valuable person wherever you spend the day. When I went into medicine, it was implicitly communicated to women that if you take a seat in medical school you are expected to use your medical degree in the workplace. Fortunately, both women and men are now able to cycle in and out of a career. Because work and life expectancy has expanded, there is usually ample time to re-enter the workplace when children are older—although you may miss the chance to move ahead on an ambitious career path. Life is all about choices.

The whole process of re-entry is getting much more attention. Today there are organizations dedicated to helping women return to work when children are older, and to getting women up to speed with new computer skills and whatever else they've missed. Volunteer work can also be valuable while you're home. Most volunteer organizations offer structured assignments where you can learn marketable skills.

I'm afraid I'll be bored if I stay home. How can I be sure?

Some people are bored and/or anxious. Although some love being home with an infant, others miss the challenge of work. That does not mean that they love their baby any less than mothers who stay home. Some parents feel it is more important to be with the children when they are older and need help and support with homework and after-school activities. Some want to be home to monitor teenagers.

If you have made the choice to stay home with your infant but are feeling trapped or depressed, get outside. Make friends with other mothers or fathers in the park. Sign up for swim classes. Join an online parenting group. Sign up for a gym or take an online course while the baby sleeps. There are lots of activities that you can incorporate into your life with baby.

Remember, we're all different. Florence was a career person who found (to her shock) that she loved staying home. She discovered another part of herself. I had the opposite experience. I loved being with my babies, but I was not good at indoor activities with them. I was better off working. Once they were older and could play sports, I was in my element. We all have our strengths.

How much maternity leave does it take to bond with the baby before going back to work?

You're embarking on a lifelong journey with your child, and bonding takes place every day. The most important part of maternity leave is a chance for you to recover from childbirth and get breastfeeding off to a good start. Research suggests the longer the maternity leave, the better it is for the mother's health.

Don't other countries offer better maternity benefits?

Unfortunately, the United States lags far behind other advanced industrial countries in maternity benefits. Women in those nations get maternity leaves (mostly paid) averaging fourteen months. Canadian women are entitled to one year of paid maternity leave. A Harvard study found that of 163 countries with some form of maternity leave, U.S. maternity benefits ranked with Lesotho, Papua New Guinea, and Swaziland.

What is the usual maternity leave in the United States?

Most mothers in this country who return to work do so in three months or less, often piecing together a combination of paid maternity leave and accrued vacation time. An examination of research found that 7 percent of mothers were working one month after childbirth; 26 percent were working at two months; and 41 percent were on the job by three months. By then you are physically healed and the baby, hopefully, has a schedule. In many occupations, three months is probably the longest time you can take off from work without being out of the loop, losing a sense of what's going on, and hurting future advancement.

EASING BACK TO WORK

I'm on maternity leave and feel so anxious about going back to my job, but we need the money. Do other women feel this way?

In my experience, most mothers feel torn when returning to work. Intermittent leave provisions under the Family and Medical Leave Act of 1995 (FMLA) allow you to ease in, first returning part time and gradually increasing your hours. However, a doctor must certify this schedule is necessary. Talk to your obstetrician about this.

How can I approach my employer about pumping breast milk at work?

Research this in advance. First ask other female employees who have young children whether they pumped on site, and what solutions they found. Some companies have a special room in place for pumping. Or you can go to human resources and ask about the company policy or to your superior. In some states, companies are required by law to provide a place to pump.

I'd like to spend more time with my baby. Is it risky to ask my boss for flextime?

It depends on how family friendly your employer is, the state of the economy, and how fragile your work situation is. If you're in an intense, competitive field, lots of bosses put you in a different category. Some call this the "Mommy Track." You may not be overtly marginalized, but before you know it, you are no longer in on the big decisions. If you refuse to travel or work late, you may be penalized. Ask if anyone else is getting flextime (or got it in the past). Today more and more companies are looking favorably toward flextime arrangements. The environment has changed for the better, but there is no guarantee.

I used to be very organized and on top of things, but since I had my baby I can't seem to get out the door in the morning. Any suggestions?

This is a very common post-baby phenomenon. Your life has changed, and you're not just taking care of yourself in the morning. There's more planning that needs to be done the night before. For example, if you have to drop the baby off at day care, have a travel bag all packed and ready, so all you have to do is add milk. Keep the bag near the door. If you lay out the baby's clothes (and yours) the night before and set up the coffee maker, you'll be calmer in the morning. The baby is likely to sense that and be less fussy. It also helps to take enough relaxed time together with the baby before you leave the house.

My spouse is very supportive of my working, but since I went back to work we're fighting all the time. What should I do?

It's the stress of juggling so many responsibilities at once. Often one party is not quite picking up their share. But sometimes it's just too much and everyone's circuits are overloaded. When both of you come home from work, you may be tired, hungry, and starving for down time. Instead, the nanny leaves or goes upstairs. Or you've picked up a tired, fussy baby at day care. You want to spend time with the baby, but the competing needs of household, marriage, and your own body make this a difficult time. Some couples take turns cooking or one goes for a run while the other plays with the baby. Try not to escalate tensions during this tricky evening period, as babies easily pick up the vibes and may add to it by screaming.

CHILD CARE OPTIONS

What choice is best—day care, nanny, mother-in-law, or babysitters?

Two out of three American children under a year old are cared for by someone other than their parent. In 50 percent of cases, the caretaker is a grandparent or other family member. Day care, nannies, or babysitters account for most of the rest. The best choice is a personal decision. It depends on your budget, the resources available in your area, your work schedule, the location of your work site, and the proximity of family members willing to pitch in and help. Some grandparents have jobs themselves. One mother chose day care because a quality facility was located nearby and her friends, whose babies were in the same day care center, recommended it. Another family hired a nanny because they didn't want to deal with picking up and delivering the baby or scrambling for a sitter when the baby was sick and needed to stay home.

Some parents are biased against their baby being cared for in someone else's home (known as family day care), yet others like a small setting with just a few children. Some don't like day care centers; others like the stimulation day care can provide. Some feel a nanny isolates the baby or worry the child will fall behind due to lack of stimulation. All these considerations are intangibles. The number of children you have may dictate which solution is possible. It's a challenge to dress and pack up more than one for day care.

At what age is it okay to put the baby in day care?

Ideally wait until your baby is at least eight weeks old because babies are immunologically vulnerable before then. Interferon, which is one of the immunological tools to fight infection, is less effective earlier. In addition, before eight weeks it's hard to tell whether a baby has a fever due to something minor like a cold or is seriously ill. The doctor should see any baby this age with a fever.

Will my baby feel insecure if she goes to day care as young as eight weeks?
Babies do well at day care when there is consistency and a good staff-to-baby ratio. A clean environment with age-appropriate stimulation and warm, loving providers who frequently hold and touch the children ensure your baby will have a good start in life. Quality day care has been time-tested and is a good option.

How to Choose a Day Care Center
Ask these questions:
- Is it licensed? Small ones may not be licensed.
- What is the cost?
- What are the hours? Pick-up times may be as early as 5:00 p.m., which can be tough for most working parents.
- When is it closed? Holidays when you have to work?
- Is the location convenient to home or office? Which is most important to you?
- What is the sick policy? Most centers have a protocol outlining which symptoms require children to stay home.
- What is the ratio of staff to children? AAP recommends a ratio of one staff member for every three babies.

- What's the staff turnover? Ask parents and the staff. This is a huge factor because babies need consistent providers for security.
- What's the age of the staff? You don't want everyone to be young and inexperienced. But you also want people who are young enough to have the mental and physical stamina to keep up with your crawling or newly walking baby..
- What's the facility's reputation? Get references from other parents.
- Do staff welcome unannounced observations and visits?
- What activities are offered? Are they age appropriate? Are they creative and interesting? Do children go outside and get exercise and fresh air? What equipment do they have?
- Are phone calls allowed? You need to be able to reach the center at times.
- What are their food policies? If your child has food allergies, will he be protected? Are junk food and juice on the menu?
- How do staff members interact with your child? Are they warm?

How does the total picture add up? How bad is traffic to and from the center? A beautiful day care center near your office may be ideal, unless traffic and parking are major hassles. On a holiday when you are home (or if you're out of town on business), day care near work may not be convenient. Be sure to visit the facility before you sign up. Don't assume it must be okay just because it's licensed.

Do babies get sick more often in day care?
Absolutely. They catch infections from each other. The upside is that baby will start to build some immunity after two months and be healthier for it. Factor into your plans the reality that if you choose day care, you're going to have to take more time off.

Does day care put my baby at higher risk for ear infection?
If your baby has a tendency for ear infections, he'll have more of them. It depends on anatomy and the Eustachian tubes.

My baby stays at home with one babysitter. Is she at a disadvantage by not getting stimulation babies get in day care?
Before two to three years of age it probably doesn't matter. After that she needs to learn to share and other basic skills. You or the babysitter can arrange for play dates at your home or elsewhere to provide socialization opportunities. If she has lots of siblings, she's getting all the socialization she needs at home.

Is it better to keep the baby in day care five days a week (even though I'm home two of those days) to avoid a disruption in her schedule?
There's no right answer. Young children do better with a regular schedule. Changes in schedule make separation harder for them. But you have to weigh that consideration against the additional "mommy time" you and the baby would have. My vote is for more time with your child.

If my baby is sick, should I send him to day care that day?
It depends on the illness. A baby that has fever, diarrhea, conjunctivitis, or is vomiting won't be allowed in day care.

Rashes must be diagnosed. For example, an allergic rash, once treated, is not contagious. Once the doctor says, "Give him Benadryl," for an allergic reaction, he can go back to day care. If it's just a stuffy nose or cough, you have to use your judgment because these can last weeks.

The key is to know what the child has. If it's just a cold and he's a day or two into it, it may be fine to go back.

What should I consider if I want to use a family day care arrangement where the provider has her own baby?

Family day care can be great, but it is not regulated the way regular day care is. Be sure to get references. If the person in charge has her own child present, one issue is, "Does her child get more attention and preferential treatment? Is there a conflict of interest?" In one family day care situation I know of, the children don't go outside because the caregiver can't manage it. You may not want an older child inside all day long.

HIRING A NANNY AND/OR BABYSITTERS

What's the best way to find a good nanny?

Word of mouth from people who have used the nanny is always best. There are also all sorts of nanny services. The agency vets candidates, but that doesn't mean you shouldn't vet, too. You need to get verbal references not just written ones. Pick up the phone and talk to the parent. People hesitate to say things in writing that could lead to a libel suit. If the candidate left the job, find out why.

Some people refer to postings at their place of worship or newspaper or online ads for agencies. Pediatricians don't give recommendations because it's inappropriate. We're in no position to evaluate the candidate.

How can I evaluate a potential nanny?

Ask her to come to your house for an interview. Is she on time? If not, don' t hire her. My husband and I violated that rule a few times, much to our regret. Is she clean and well kept? Is she warm and welcoming to the baby? Does she have a smile on her face and talk and play with the baby? Get a sense of what she's looking for and why she does this job. If it's just because she needs the money, that's not good enough. Nannies should love children and really want to do this. How long does she plan to work for you? Is this temporary while her husband looks for a job? What transportation will she use? A ten-year-old car subject to breakdowns can be a disaster. I'm an expert at weeding out candidates because I've made my share of mistakes.

Focus on the person's experience. You might ask a few hypothetical questions like "What would you do if the baby ate the scouring powder?" Make sure the person can tolerate isolation, too. Often young people don't do well with that. They'll either be on the cell phone all the time or watching TV. Figure out in advance what your expectations are, make a list, and go over it with the applicant. One mom's top priority is "I want my kid to be loved." If you want light housekeeping, make sure candidates know it's part of the job. People who are organized like to plan ahead, but the applicant may want to start work right away. Some parents hire the nanny before they actually need her to avoid losing her to another family.

How do I know if I'm asking too much or too little of the nanny?

If you require a host of housekeeping duties, the baby will suffer. On the other hand, beware of a candidate who seems too chummy during the interview. The nanny is not your friend. You want to be able to tell her what you want her to do or the arrangement will fall apart. Some parents, especially young parents, have trouble taking charge.

I'm afraid my baby will love the nanny more than me. How can I stop that from happening?

In the short term you can't stop it. The person who delivers care and cuddling will be number one. But the nanny won't be there forever. This is one of the sacrifices you make. If you feed the baby in the morning, evening, and the middle of the night, the baby will bond with you. But sometimes the baby will show preference for the nanny. This is usually temporary.

How can I avoid revolving nannies?

Some couples switch nannies every year (or even more frequently), which is hard on the baby and on you. Try to view the nanny as a "third partner," rather than someone to be ordered around. Try a review every five or six months where you can say, "You're doing a good job, but Bobby needs more floor time" or "This is how you can improve." Give the nanny a chance to speak up, too, by asking, "Is there anything that's bothering you?" Maybe the nanny feels a particular rule is unreasonable.

What's better—a grandparent or a babysitter?

Forty percent of grandparents are regular caregivers for grandchildren living nearby. In most cases, no sitter is going to love your baby (and keep an eagle eye on her) like a grandparent will. In fact, a 2008 Johns Hopkins study found that children whose grandparents were their caregivers had roughly half the injuries of those under other types of care. This is extra important when you consider that injuries are the number one cause of death of children in this country. But it's critical that the grandparent is the one who volunteers. Some grandparents don't want to be a parent again. Let grandparents be who they are, and don't guilt trip them. If they want to babysit, great, but it should be on their terms.

In certain cultures such as Indian, Hispanic, Arab, and many Asian cultures, family members naturally take on this responsibility; in others they do not. I see Asian women who leave their own homes for weeks and months to go live with their children and help with a grandchild. That certainly is not typical in American culture.

Is it important to have my baby in a play group?

Play groups at one year or less are more for the social benefit of parents, but that's important, too. If you have social outlets and are happy, the baby will be happy. It's good for a nanny to get out, as well, and maybe befriend another nanny in a play group.

COMMUNICATING WITH CAREGIVERS

How can I get off on the right foot with the nanny I'm hiring?

First, set rules and communicate expectations upfront to prevent problems. Make it crystal clear what is and is not okay. When can she watch TV? Only at certain times, such as when the baby is sleeping? Is your policy "no cell phone," except for emergencies or communication with you? Are friends or boyfriends allowed in your home? For many of us, it's hard to say what we expect. It almost seems insulting when we say it. But if you're not clear, the person can wind up talking on the cell phone all the time because she wasn't told not to.

What if the nanny breaks a rule you set?

Address the issue immediately and be firm. You might say, "Remember we talked about 'no friends in my house'? Please don't do this again." You don't want to be too strict or you won't hold onto anyone, but you do need agreed-upon rules to be followed.

My baby never seems tired in the evening when he's with the babysitter. We think she's letting him sleep too long during day. How can we confirm this?

Short of asking or popping in on her, it's her word. It's tricky because in the first year babies vary so much. It could be unfair to the sitter. But you can always say, "The baby won't go to sleep at night. Let's try shortening her afternoon nap." You might also make an unannounced visit at a time the baby should have awakened from the nap, or ask a friend or neighbor to do it for you. Remember, babies can't talk. There's no way of monitoring.

What's the best way to complain about something a day care center is doing?

Most centers have a director, who is the person to whom you'd present your complaint. For instance, if the shades are pulled down and it's boiling hot on a 100-degree day, that's unhealthy and you should mention it to the director.

How can I get my mother-in-law to follow my rules for the baby, rather than hers, without alienating her?

This can be a loaded situation, whether it's your mother-in-law, your own mother, or another relative. Her view is that she raised her children just fine and her way is best. She may not be aware of all the changes in bringing up baby that have occurred due to new research, new developments, and new health issues. If this is going to be a regular arrangement, as painful and awkward as it is, the best idea is to have a discussion with Grandma before she takes on babysitting. It's harder to do that with a family member than with someone you've hired, but try something like, "We've thought about this as a couple, and this is how we feel about the baby finishing her bottle (or about the length of daytime naps)."

I've seen cases where a grandparent babysits during the week and stuffs the child with food. The mom is indebted to

Talking Together

Most couples *do* discuss whether or not mom will return to work. What they don't anticipate is the reality. Flexibility counts because you can't always predict how you will feel. One new mother went back to work after three months but missed her daughter so much that she left her job. Talk about the home support your spouse will provide when you return to work. It's more productive and less stressful to negotiate before you go back, rather than put it off and find yourself too overwhelmed to problem solve.

Discuss instructions you want the nanny or other caregiver to follow in order to avoid contradicting each other. It's important to stay on the same page. You also have to anticipate that nannies call in sick or get stuck in traffic jams and that day care centers can close. Kids may freak out when they have to go to another day care because it's a totally new environment. Play "what if" together and figure out a plan just in case. Some companies offer back up child care. Maybe one of you can take the baby to the office, if necessary. One couple took turns staying home from work part of each day when their six-month-old had a bad ear infection and was a mess. It's tough when you both work full time, but there may be options you haven't thought about before. If you're staying home, be realistic about time off for yourself and discuss baby sitter relief. I know of one case where a mom who works part time and a mom who stays home share a sitter.

Sometimes expectations about double paychecks fall apart if mom decides she would rather stay home and leave her job. One parent may want a live-in nanny while the other prefers day care. Discussing such issues may seem basic, but these are the problems that lead to bickering and sniping at each other. What counts is that both of you express your feelings and decide how the issue adds up.

her but is terrified the baby will wind up obese. This is a common sticking point. Research shows that infants cared for by a grandparent weigh more and are started on solid foods earlier (a risk factor for obesity) than those cared for by a parent. Otherwise, this is an ideal babysitting arrangement.

Of course you want to be diplomatic, and clear in your own mind about what you want. Another option is "blame the doctor." For example, if your mother insists on feeding table food to the baby, but he's supposed to eat pureed food, tell her, "The pediatrician insists on pureed food only." If she objects, reply, "I hear what you're saying, but I have to follow the doctor's instructions."

DIFFICULT DECISIONS

"I cried for days before I went back to work. My son wouldn't take the bottle and I was terrified he'd starve in day care," recalls one mother. If you stay home, you'll agonize about other problems. It's hard to be a parent whatever you do, and you can count on a long period of adjustment. Just bear in mind that these early days will fly by more quickly than you imagine, and somehow you will have found solutions. The time will come when you're asking, "What happened to my baby? He's grown too fast."

CHAPTER 15

Marriage—
Maintaining the Relationship

This chapter covers:

- Keeping your relationship strong
- Resuming sex
- Resuscitation tips for your marriage
- Post-baby couple social life

Your new baby is a treasure that can bring new depth and meaning to your marriage. But becoming a parent also casts the two of you into a world of stressful change. The challenge is not to immerse yourselves so totally in the parenting experience that the air is sucked out of the house. The baby isn't the only one who needs nurturing. Relationships can be fragile and complicated. Although you and your partner may be excited about the new family addition, the initial euphoria can quickly turn to hurt and resentment if the household begins to center around the baby. The healthiest families are those that include children as part of the family, rather than the focus of it. Good marriages require attention, and that must start from day one as parents.

These questions and answers can help you identify issues that are likely to arise and figure out ways to protect intimacy.

STAYING CLOSE

We're constantly exhausted and seem to have no time for each other. How can we reconnect?

Exhaustion goes with parenting. Time together without the baby will not happen unless you make it happen. Instead of feeling guilty about couple time, look at it as an investment for the entire family. If your marriage stays rich, the entire family benefits.

Line up some reliable babysitters and arrange regular dates on the calendar to be alone together without interruption, even if it's just for an hour or two. Maybe you can hire someone at the baby's day care center once a week to enjoy a night out. Says one mom, "Your marriage will die if you don't plan a date outside the house. It's important to stick to your date schedule because otherwise life can get monotonous and you get resentful." A date might consist of dinner out, grocery shopping, a walk, a movie and hand holding, or you might have to combine being together with a workout at the gym on Saturday.

I feel we're not as close as we used to be because we never talk about anything but the baby.
It's important to remain interested in the world and other parts of your lives together. Try to stay abreast of issues at home and abroad by reading the newspaper or the news online. Read a book, even if it's a few pages at a time when you can relax for a brief break. Talk to neighbors and friends and be interested in others. Although it is fun to talk about the baby, if that is all you discuss, your lives may start to seem narrow. I have seen couples bore each other to distraction with the minutiae of life with baby. If one of you is working, that partner may want to decompress at home and discuss a work issue before getting to the diaper diaries. Just because you are now a parent doesn't mean you have stopped being a person and a citizen.

When we go out, my wife is obsessed with our eight-week-old baby and has no appetite. She can't wait to get back home. Is there anything I can do about this?
Maybe you can figure out close-to-home dates that will make her feel more secure. I once saw a TV series where a

creative husband came up with the idea of picnicking on the deck with takeout food while the baby slept. In such cases, the agreement should be that although you're right there, you're going to focus only on each other. Parents often worry when they're away from their infants, but some take longer than others to separate.

If one of you refuses to ever leave the baby, it can become a problem if it bothers the other. Compromise and open discussion are the best ways to resolve such an issue. I have seen new parents become obsessed with their baby's safety. Professional counseling is in order if the result is dissension in the marriage.

Our relationship is good, but we argue a lot about picking up the baby and feeding problems. Is this natural?

No couple I've seen agrees on everything. Baby tasks get negotiated just like washing dishes and taking out the garbage. Since you both made the baby, the tasks need to be shared. If one person is working and the other stays home, the tasks may not be divided fifty-fifty. Bickering about night feedings or changing dirty diapers can escalate into large disagreements, so try to make an equitable plan from the start—and re-evaluate as you go along.

RESUMING SEX

When is it okay to have sex again?

If you've had a vaginal delivery with an episiotomy, you probably aren't going to ask this question for a while, although your spouse may. You may feel like a Mack truck has passed through your vaginal canal. But eventually, hormones settle down, wounds heal, and desire does return.

A Caesarian section involves major surgery and the abdomen needs time to heal. Obstetricians usually say sex can resume in four to six weeks, but obviously this can vary, depending on the pace of recovery and other factors.

The important point is that physical intimacy is part of a healthy relationship. If your partner is clamoring for attention, get busy in the bedroom. Hugging, kissing, and touching are key partial substitutes until your body is ready for more.

I feel fat and my breasts are leaking milk. I don't feel very attractive. How can I make myself more appealing to my husband?

Your body image can take a beating after childbirth. Your breasts and stomach are big, and other parts of your body are stretched. I've seen even beautiful women feel ugly at this time. This won't last forever. Your body image will improve with time, although it may take effort and exercise. See Chapter 16 for ideas on getting started. Your pre-pregnancy clothes may not fit yet, but filling in with something new can also give you a lift. Or you might even try a new haircut. Such little things can build confidence, and confidence is sexy.

Does it matter that neither one of us feels like having sex because we're exhausted all the time?

Physical intimacy, which comes in many forms, is what distinguishes this relationship from all others. You are not solely business partners or friends (although you may be that, too). You used to be lovers. The best recipe for a long, happy relationship is one which includes mental, emotional, and physical intimacy. Where sex was once spontaneous and urgent, you may now need to be more intentional and plan. But neglect sex at the peril of your marriage.

Post-Baby Resuscitation Tips for Your Marriage
- Say thank you to your partner for little chores.
- Tell your partner how glad you are to see him/her when either of you get home from work.
- Instead of complaining or nagging, have a quiet conversation when the household is settled.
- Remember to laugh and have fun together.
- If you don't feel like having sex, remember hugging, kissing, or cuddling are good alternatives.
- Be conscious of touching each other. A pat goes a long way. One new mom made a point of caressing the back of her husband's neck as they sat watching TV.
- Don't neglect your partner no matter how needy your little offspring is.
- Avoid snapping by getting enough rest.
- Allow change to happen. A new baby will change your relationship. Go with it and help shape it.
- Don't let third parties—including relatives, friends, or other well-meaning individuals—ruin your new family with unwanted advice
- Let your new baby be part of your life, rather than crafting a new life around the baby.

My husband wants sex and the doctor says it's okay for me, but sex is the last thing on my mind. I feel like a used washing machine. What should I do?

It's natural not to feel sexy when you still can't sit down and the last time you slept was . . . when was it? If your husband isn't doing as much to help as you'd like and you resent it, that's another damper. Try to explain your reservations to your partner. He may be patient to a point, but be sensitive to his needs, too. It is not just loss of sex, but loss of emotional intimacy that can lead to a parched relationship.

My wife hasn't lost the baby weight and never seems to dress up anymore. How can I help her?

Be patient and kind, but encourage her to get herself together once she has healed somewhat and breastfeeding is established. Take her out! A few compliments can go a long way in helping her regain her confidence.

It's hard for me to see my wife as a lover now that she's a mommy. What do I do? We used to have a great sex life.

Creating a baby leads to changes on many fronts: new roles, new bodies, new priorities. If you are having trouble resuming your sex life, talk to a professional. I have seen many marriages crumble as lovers morphed into parents and the romance was left in the delivery room.

Is my spouse having an affair at work or am I just paranoid? I think a lot of men have affairs at this time.

You may start to feel isolated and left out if you are home all day with the baby. Get back in the mix as best you can. If you are worried your husband will stray at this time, you need to share your fears and concerns with him.

RESURRECTING YOUR COUPLE SOCIAL LIFE

I feel like we have no friends. Everything's centered on work and the baby. How can we change the balance?

A social life with other couples, especially those who have young children, provides important support for your marriage. Research suggests that the more friends you share as a couple, the less likely you are to divorce. Positive couple friends provide fun, information, and support, particularly when they are in the same stage of the lifecycle as you. They're experiencing (or have recently gone through) the same situations. You can learn how they coped when day

Talking Together

Try to negotiate parenting disagreements early because parenting challenges only get more complicated and intense as children grow. Out-of-sync expectations and preferences left unaddressed lead to bickering, resentment, withheld sex, and marital discord. Beware of undermining, criticizing, or competing with each other, as some couples do. One two-career couple argues about their level of activity on weekends. He often wants to go out and visit family and friends with the baby. She usually likes to stay home and play with the baby to recover from the work week and because the baby cries constantly in the car, making car trips stressful. The goal is to respect differences, find a compromise, and realize there is no one right answer in most cases. Things change when each of you believes your needs are recognized and your voice is heard. Couple friends can be helpful here, too. You can watch (or ask) what they do in similar situations and cherry pick ideas that might work for your relationship.

Brainstorm how to collaborate, as in "I'll do X, and you do Y." A husband who must work long hours during the week can help out more on weekends to give his wife a break. Maybe you take turns picking up the baby at day care. Many studies show that having a child strains most marriages and results in a decline in marital satisfaction. If conflict seems to be creeping into your marriage since the birth of the baby, seek professional counseling sooner rather than later to referee these important discussions.

care kept sending the baby home sick. They can recommend babysitters. They can even serve as role models for how to deal with parenting conflicts—or as examples of what *not* to do.

Do we always have to take the baby on vacation with us?
Some parents want their children with them all the time, and others want and need a break alone together. This is a personal decision. Traveling with young children can be more trouble than it is worth, even with a nanny.

Travel was a big part of our relationship before the baby. Are there trips where we can bring baby along or do we have to give this up?
The parents I see travel all over the world with their children. The risk for babies, especially those under two months of age, is infection. See Chapter 9 for information on traveling with your baby.

MARRIAGE CAN BE TRICKY BUSINESS

You fell in love and produced an offspring. Maybe you waited a few years after marrying to start a family. Or maybe the baby came before the marriage certificate. Either way, "and baby makes three" changes the dynamic of the household. Remember that a baby is part of the family, not the center of it. Each member is equally important. Your relationship must be nourished in order for you both to be whole for your child.

CHAPTER 16

Caring for Yourself— How to Take Your Life Back

This chapter covers:

- Postpartum healing
- Contraception
- Baby blues and postpartum depression
- Losing weight and exercise
- Socializing

You've gone through pregnancy and childbirth and are now readjusting to the enormous life changes that a baby brings. The stress of new responsibilities and the non-stop nature of parenting an infant is harder work than you ever imagined. You may have some negative feelings about all these shifts, and it is important to acknowledge them. As one new mother puts it, "Why didn't my mom tell me?! All she talked about was the joy."

Your body has also experienced an extraordinary journey. Although you may have enjoyed being pregnant, you may long to return to your previous shape. Some women's bodies seem to stretch out to accommodate the growing baby, and then snap back into shape like a rubber band after childbirth. Others are not so fortunate and can remain overstretched. You also have healing to do internally. And you may be riding an emotional roller coaster as your hormones return to a pre-pregnancy state. Your body needs care and attention whether you had a vaginal delivery or a Caesarian section.

These questions and answers focus on the wear and tear on mind and body at this time and help guide you to a healthy recovery.

PHYSICAL ISSUES

What does the term "postpartum" really mean?
The postpartum period is generally considered the time needed for the mother's body to heal after childbirth. The assumption has been that it takes about six weeks; however, research now suggests that recovery from childbirth can take longer.

When should I have a postpartum checkup?
This visit with your obstetrician is usually recommended at four to six weeks after delivery. But contact your obstetrician right away if you experience any unusual problems, such as excessive vaginal blood loss, foul smelling vaginal discharge, fever, or severe breast pain. Write down any questions you have and bring the list along to your visit. Birth control should be discussed at this checkup, whether or not you're breastfeeding.

How much vaginal bleeding is normal after giving birth?
Expect a heavy flow of blood in the first few days. This should decrease day by day and eventually stop. Be aware that too much physical activity too fast can cause bleeding again. If you feel lightheaded or the blood flow increases, tell your obstetrician right away.

I have pain from an episiotomy. How should I treat it?
An episiotomy is a procedure that may be necessary to enlarge the vaginal opening to ease passage of the baby during delivery. Stitches close the cut after the birth. Cool witch hazel pads used as panty liners can help relieve discomfort. You may also want to sit on a "doughnut pillow" for a while and/or take the painkillers your doctor prescribed. An episiotomy tends to hurt most after the birth of a first baby.

I've heard that you can have anemia after giving birth. Why, and what can be done about it?

After childbirth, heavy bleeding and/or poor diet can cause the red blood cell count to fall abnormally low. Anemia is closely monitored by the obstetrician, who usually keeps the mother on prenatal vitamins if she is breastfeeding. Any new mom with anemia should eat foods rich in iron, such as red meat, spinach, broccoli, or foods cooked in an iron skillet. (The iron in the pan passes into the food.)

I have continual back pain since my baby arrived. Is that a side effect of delivery?

Many of the aches and pains you experienced during your third trimester of pregnancy disappear after giving birth, but not all of them. Hormones released during pregnancy caused changes in several parts of your body. For example, the bones of the pelvis opened up to allow room for the baby to pass through. It may take a while for stretched bones, muscles, and connective tissue to return to normal, a process that can be painful. If you received an epidural for anesthesia during delivery, you may experience back pain later. If back pain persists, report it to your doctor. It could be an orthopedic or other medical problem.

Why are hemorrhoids common after you give birth?

Veins in areas such as the rectum and lower legs have valves to keep blood flowing back to the heart, rather than pooling in the legs. Babies can weigh enough during pregnancy to put pressure on these valves, damage them, and cause blood in the veins to back up rather than flow freely. This can lead to varicose veins in the legs or hemorrhoids, which are swollen veins in the anus or rectum. Both can be painful.

Is there a risk of blood clots after childbirth?

It is important to get up and about after childbirth (or any period of inactivity) to prevent blood from pooling in the lower extremities and causing clots to form. Even mothers in pain from an episiotomy are told to walk around. Some people are prone to blood clots, such as those who took birth control pills before pregnancy or who take them after the baby is born.

I was never constipated until I gave birth. Why?

Constipation may occur after childbirth for a couple of reasons. If you've had an episiotomy and are in pain, you may hesitate to bear down to eliminate. For this reason, your doctor may give you a stool softener. Constipation can also be a side effect of pain medications you take after delivery. Try to get your intestines moving again because the longer you go without a bowel movement, the harder the stool becomes. Fresh fruit and vegetables, lots of fluids, and walking will help.

Is there a danger of incontinence after childbirth?

Childbirth can wreak havoc on parts of women's bodies, although young women recover quickly. Both fecal and urinary stress incontinence, usually temporary, can occur when you sneeze or cough. Once you regain some of your pelvic muscle tone, these symptoms hopefully disappear.

What are Kegel exercises?

Pelvic muscle tone can return passively on its own, but a little active assistance from you in the form of Kegel exercises can speed things along. Ask your obstetrician to show you how to use these and other toning exercises to tighten up the sphincters for urine and stool, as well as the other pelvic floor muscles.

Why do some women need C-sections?

Any time the mother or baby's health is in immediate jeopardy, obstetricians will move to deliver the baby in the fastest, least stressful way possible—by C-section. Doctors may elect C-section for other reasons, as well. For example, the baby may be too big to fit through the birth canal. Or the position of the placenta (the tissue that delivers nourishment and blood supply from mother to baby in utero) may raise the risk of placenta rupture and hemorrhage in a vaginal delivery. If the mother had a previous C-section, more and more obstetricians elect to do repeat C-sections rather than vaginal deliveries. The concern is rupturing of the uterus at the site of the old C-section scar.

How is C-section recovery different from recovery from vaginal delivery?

A C-section is major abdominal surgery. The incision must heal and close, which can be painful and take time. As with any surgery, there is risk of infection and other complications. New mothers who have had C-sections generally stay in the hospital a few more days than women who deliver vaginally.

What can I do about my C-Section scar?

I usually tell people to wait before taking action on any scar because the passage of time can make a big difference. Scars often fade all by themselves. Some doctors recommend vitamin E cream to minimize C-section scarring. Be sure to apply sun block to the scar if you are back in your bikini because sunburn makes it worse. If you have the tendency to form keloids, red raised fibrous tissue that builds up at the site of a healing scar, you may want to consult a plastic surgeon down the road.

When should I expect to menstruate again after childbirth?

Once postpartum bleeding stops for good, it may be several months before your normal menstrual cycle resumes, especially if you are breastfeeding. But do not think that you're protected from pregnancy if you haven't yet had a period. Many babies have been born due to this false assumption. See Chapter 15 for information on resuming your sex life.

Do I need contraception when I am breastfeeding my baby?

Yes, you do. Speak with your obstetrician right after delivery about when to resume contraception. If you have been using a barrier device such as the Nuva Ring or a diaphragm, you may need to be refitted. Although you may not menstruate for a while, especially if you are breastfeeding, you do not want to discover that the absence of your period is the start of another pregnancy—unless you do!

Why did I get stretch marks and what can I do about them?

Stretch marks can appear when collagen in the second layer of skin (dermis) is suddenly stretched, as in pregnancy. After delivery and subsequent weight loss, these marks are reduced in number and size, but some may remain. Not everyone gets stretch marks, and there seems to be a genetic component. Many over-the-counter products are touted for removal of stretch marks, but I do not know of any that work well. If stretch marks persist after you have done all you can to lose weight and tone up, you may wish to consult a plastic surgeon or dermatologist. Stretch marks are only a cosmetic problem and are not harmful.

I sweat and get hot flashes since giving birth. Is this normal?

Following delivery, your body undergoes a hormonal upheaval that often simulates menopausal symptoms. A sudden drop in estrogen can cause major night sweats and flushing temporarily. If you're affected by a hormonal storm, be prepared. Place beside your bed a menopause tool kit, including a small handheld battery-powered fan, a towel to place under you to soak up sweat, and a spare nightgown for middle-of-the-night changes, if necessary.

I'm breastfeeding. How should I take care of my breasts?

Cracked nipples, nipple soreness, blocked milk ducts, mastitis, and other problems can occur when breastfeeding. See Chapter 2 for more information.

How can I deal with my exhaustion?

Exhaustion is one of the most common problems new parents face. Your emotions and body are fragile right now and you need to care for yourself as well as the baby. This is a time to learn to say no to chores that can wait or well-meaning friends and relatives who may want to visit when you're not up to company. Of course make it a point to sleep when the baby sleeps (even if it's a catnap). Ask for help when you need it. Maybe a friend who works at home or a family member can spend an hour or two with the baby occasionally, allowing you to take a refreshing nap. On the other hand, tell your doctor what's going on. There are medical conditions that can cause fatigue and exhaustion—such as thyroid problems, anemia, or depression—that may need treatment.

EMOTIONAL EFFECTS AND POSTPARTUM DEPRESSION

I cry all the time. Why do I feel this way when I have a healthy baby and this should be a happy time?

Mood swings tend to accompany the sudden drop in estrogen after childbirth. These swings can cause wild euphoria, sharp bursts of anger, or sudden tearful meltdowns. Baby blues, which usually disappear in a week or two, affect 50 to 80 percent of new mothers. Try to catch up on sleep whenever you can to help regain your emotional equilibrium. Fatigue worsens these normal mood shifts. Swings should be easier to control once you understand and are aware of them.

What's the difference between baby blues and postpartum depression?

The temporary emotional upheaval that may occur after delivery is quite different from postpartum depression, which is a serious form of depression. Postpartum depression is characterized by stronger, longer lasting symptoms than baby blues. Once recognized, it should be treated right away by a mental health professional. In addition to mood swings, anxiety, crying, and other signs, women with postpartum depression may have thoughts of harming the baby or themselves or be indifferent to the child. They may also suffer from insomnia or excess sleep, loss of appetite or overeating; the simplest chores may seem overwhelming.

What causes postpartum depression?

We don't know for certain, but hormonal changes after childbirth may bring on symptoms. A family history (or your own history) of depression probably puts you at higher risk. Stressful events such as a death or illness in the family or the mother's return to work after maternity leave may contribute as well.

How is postpartum depression treated?

Treatment may include therapy and/or medication. If you think you are suffering from postpartum depression, tell your obstetrician and pediatrician. They can help you seek medical care from a mental health professional. Support groups can also be useful. The National Institute of Mental Health (NIMH) estimates that postpartum depression affects anywhere from 10 to 15 percent of new mothers. It is a medical condition, not an indication of failure as a mother. Without help, the baby, your marriage, and you are at risk. You can call 1-866-615-6464 (National Institute of Mental Health) to be connected with a twenty-four-hour crisis hotline and for referrals to mental health professionals in your area.

WEIGHT LOSS AND NUTRITION

How much weight is usually lost right after giving birth?

The average weight gain during pregnancy is anywhere from twenty-five to thirty-five pounds. Most women lose twelve-and-a-half to fourteen pounds after delivery. That leaves some excess weight that should come off with time, breastfeeding, exercise, and a sensible, healthy diet.

I'm breastfeeding. How many calories should I eat?

Generally a nursing mother should eat 1500 to 1800 calories a day. However, bear in mind that the calorie requirement depends on body type, metabolism, and activity level. You may need more or fewer calories to reach your desired weight. It is extremely important to eat healthy and drink lots of fluids to successfully breastfeed. Be patient. It takes time for some weight and shape changes to occur.

I can't seem to lose this baby weight. How come actresses on TV lose it in a month?

You would probably do the same if you had a personal trainer working out with you every day and a personal chef to make sure your diet is perfect. The rest of us need to be disciplined about diet, exercise, and getting enough sleep. Give it time.

I have an awfully big appetite now that I'm breast-feeding. Is there a connection?

Breastfeeding burns about 200 to 500 extra calories a day, and your body needs fuel. You may also burn extra calories at night with night feedings and all the moving around involved in baby care. Beware of overestimating the latter, however.

Are there certain vitamins I should take now?

Breastfeeding moms should continue the prenatal vitamins they took during pregnancy because they are losing nutrients through breast milk. If you are iron deficient due to extra blood loss during delivery, your obstetrician may put you on a therapeutic dose of supplemental iron. A therapeutic dose, which treats iron deficiency, is far more potent than a maintenance dose to *prevent* deficiency. Even if you're bottle feeding, your doctor may tell you to continue on a multivitamin until your strength returns and you are eating a normal diet.

I heard that breastfeeding can cause calcium depletion. How can I avoid that?

Continue taking prenatal vitamins, drink milk if you can, and eat foods rich in calcium such as dairy products and broccoli.

Are there any foods I should avoid while breastfeeding?

Too much caffeine, chocolate, or rich spicy foods in your diet may have an effect on your baby. Excessive caffeine can cause jitteriness and irritability in infants. Moderation is the key. But keep in mind that babies often have gas and can be fussy. In my experience, too many mothers tend to blame gas on their own diet when that is not the case.

What do I need to eat to maintain my milk supply?

A balanced healthy diet is important, but fluids and rest are the most important elements in maintaining a good milk supply.

Can I diet while I'm breastfeeding?

If you eat healthy foods, there is no reason to diet. You need energy to care for the baby and you must replenish the nutrients used in pregnancy, childbirth, and breastfeeding.

I usually take a medication for depression. Can I take it while breastfeeding?

Some antidepressants are approved for breastfeeding mothers, but be sure to clear the medication with your obstetrician and pediatrician. We don't know whether many psychiatric medications have long-term effects on the baby.

EXERCISE

When is it safe to start exercising again?

That depends on factors such as type of delivery (vaginal or C-section), whether there were complications, whether you had an episiotomy or a vaginal tear, and most important, how you feel. Lack of sleep, trouble producing enough milk, or continuing vaginal bleeding may be factors, as well. Your obstetrician will help you determine a good starting date for your body and situation. You want to ease back into exercise routines slowly to prevent injury to recovering bone, muscle, and connective tissue.

I don't have a babysitter. How can I get to the gym?

Take turns with your husband. When he's at home, you go out to the gym. Many health clubs and gyms also have free babysitting services. Find out whether yours is one of them. Or your place of worship may have a list of babysitting volunteers.

Ask around. You can also trade with other parents, as in "You stay with my baby while I play tennis, and I'll babysit for you when you want to work out." Or call on Grandma, or even a willing neighbor as long as you don't go to the well too often.

One mom with a demanding job, and a baby in day care who is sick a lot, says, "I go to the gym at 5:00 a.m., but it isn't always possible. Sometimes I've been up during the night when he's sick and I choose extra sleep over working out." In general, however, you can put exercise on the daily to-do list and make it happen. You will be surprised at how working out can actually reduce fatigue, in addition to improving fitness and your sense of well being.

How can we work out an exercise routine together because that was an important part of our marriage before the baby arrived?

A little planning in advance can allow you both to get in a workout. For example, exercise together at home when the baby is sleeping. Buy a jogger, and all three of you can go for a run. Join a health club with day care. I have found that exercise is possible if parents are committed to it.

What sort of exercise equipment is best at home when you're on a budget?

You can walk up and down the stairs in your house or condo. Look for secondhand equipment at yard sales (or on Craigslist, E-Bay, or in the Yellow Pages). Weights are cheap. Do sit-ups and pushups, which don't require equipment. Buy some postnatal exercise books and videos or borrow them from the library. Take advantage of exercise programs on cable TV. There are some excellent DVDs with yoga and exercise programs you can do at home.

If you're housebound, you can also put on some music and dance. Anything that gets you off that couch and pumps your heart rate up is beneficial.

Postpartum Naptime Exercise

I asked international fitness expert Tracey Mallett, author of *Super Fit Mama,* to suggest exercises you can squeeze in while the baby is napping, even during brief naps. Be sure to check with your obstetrician first before trying these or any other exercises.

Tracey says, "You can make huge gains with mini cardio intervals and strength training using your own body weight for resistance when performed consistently. Always wear a good support bra and have your sneakers at hand ready to go."

Cardio Baby Fat Blast

Move from one exercise to another without a break, which is known as a cardio circuit. The duration of the circuit is seven minutes plus warm up and cool down. For a longer workout, repeat the circuit a few times.

WARM UP. Casually walk around your living room, gently circling your arms at your sides. This allows your heart rate to elevate slightly. (Two minutes)

KNEE LIFTS WITH OVERHEAD PRESS. Start with your feet hip-width apart and your arms by your sides. Reach arms overhead toward the ceiling and at the same time, alternate lifting left and right knees toward your chest. (Two minutes)

JUMP SQUAT. Start with feet hip-width apart, toes pointing forward, arms by your side. Jump up toward the ceiling, and at the same time reach your arms overhead. As you land, bend knees over your toes into a squat position with your arms by your sides. Repeat the jump as you extend the legs. *If you are unable to jump into a squat, rise onto your toes instead. Then flatten feet on floor and bend knees over toes into squat.* (Twenty seconds)

SKI STEP. Stand on one leg and bend the opposite leg behind the body. Jump off your supporting leg to the side and land on other foot. Keep jumping side to side, landing on one leg with the opposite arm extended in front of you. (Two minutes)

RUN OR MARCH AS FAST AS YOU CAN IN PLACE. (Twenty seconds)

SHUFFLE STEP. Shuffle four steps to the right and four steps to the left. Put a spring in your step and push off each leg working the butt muscles. Follow with two steps to the right and two steps to the left—again working the butt muscles. (Two minutes total for both)

MARCH IN PLACE to recover. (Twenty seconds)

Repeat the circuit two more times. If the baby wakes up after you've completed only two circuits, perform the last one later in the day when your partner gets home.

After completing three circuits in a row, cool down for two minutes by walking around the living room taking deep breaths— inhaling through the nose and exhaling through the mouth.

Cardio time: 25 minutes for three circuits, including warm up and cool down of two minutes each.

Note: Tracey also suggests loading up your MP3 player with some motivating songs at a moderate tempo to work a little harder if you wish. But always listen to your body. Never push yourself to exhaustion. While exercising you should always be able to hold a conversation. If this proves too difficult, you're working out at too high an intensity. Remember your baby needs you energized.

LOSE THE ABS FLAB

You can also reactivate those stretched-out abdominal muscles to get flatter abs back after baby, says exercise expert Tracey Mallett. Start either by lying on your back with knees bent or sitting up tall on a chair (or even while driving your car). Inhale through the nose and feel your ribcage expand as your lungs fill with air. Then as you exhale through the mouth, draw the abdominal wall in toward the spine, and you will feel your abdominal muscles contract. (Imagine you are scooping out your midsection.) For best results, repeat this exercise for ten repetitions, three times daily.

SOCIALIZING ISSUES

How can I feel like a whole person again?

Don't get stuck indoors. Go outside whenever you can and get together with people. Although you may feel as though your baby is your new best friend, life can be somewhat sterile without a good laugh with girlfriends, golf or tennis pals, other couples, and relatives. Maintaining existing friendships and family relationships and making new best friends beyond the tiniest member of the household help you regain your life post-baby.

Where can I meet other new parents?

In many parks, you can see gatherings of chatting parents with strollers. Take a chance and introduce yourself. Talk to other parents at day care. One Cambridge restaurant near my home is filled with parents, babies, and toddlers. Is there someone with a baby at the next table? Try starting a conversation. Do the same in line at the supermarket. Sometimes nannies who become friends introduce the parents they work for.

Keep an eye out for neighbors with babies. Reach out to coworkers who recently became parents—or the couple you met in prenatal classes. One mother found an online networking site of local moms who meet weekly to go to museums and other stroller-friendly places. The point is friends don't show up out of the blue. You have to be proactive. If you're shy, I assure you most new parents are in the same situation you are and will be happy to meet you.

Women need the intimacy and connection of female friends in the same situation. Other new moms may be older or younger than you, but you have so much in common. Try not to be too picky. Even if you don't feel perfectly compatible with such friends, remember that they can be very useful. As one mom puts it, "When I need to confide in someone, I call my best friend from college. But when I need input about colic, I want the mom down the road."

I have some friends who don't have children yet, and we don't have much fun together anymore. How can we recharge our relationship?

Respect that your priorities and lifestyles are out of sync right now. That doesn't mean you stop seeing them, but maybe you get together less often. Be sensitive to the fact they may not be interested in long stories about the baby. Assure them your preoccupation with the baby will eventually subside.

I've returned to work full time and I'm exhausted at the end of the day. How can we socialize when I'm worn out?

You have to prioritize. If you are working and caring for a baby, a social life may not be in the cards right now. Find other ways to maintain friendships through e-mail, walks, or having coffee. Formal dinner parties are great when you are just a couple and can study the latest celebrity chef's fish dish, but keep it simple for now.

Can I bring the baby to an adult evening occasion?

It depends. Is it a business dinner or a barbecue in the backyard? Are the hosts child-oriented or not? Some couples have brought babies to weddings (both with and without nannies). Unless you know for certain that children are welcome, it's inappropriate to just show up without checking with the hosts first. Lots of people want adult occasions to be a time they get away from their own children, and they may not want to cope with yours. For formal events such as weddings, don't ask if you haven't been told to bring along the baby. It's very awkward for the hosts to say no.

How to Spot a Baby-Friendly Restaurant

- No linen tablecloths
- Carriage and stroller lineup outside the door
- Play area when meltdown is imminent
- Nursing-friendly
- Lots of noise inside (so your baby's squall will not be noticed)
- Management doesn't grimace when you ask for a table
- Booster and high chairs available
- Smoke and alcohol blasts do not meet you at the door
- Quick service (and I do mean quick)

When is it okay to bring the baby to a restaurant for dinner?

You can always pick one of the many kid-friendly restaurants if you want to take her along. I would not bring a baby to an obviously "adults-only" restaurant. It's inappropriate to subject others out for a relaxing evening to a wailing infant.

Why are some parents I meet so competitive about their babies?

I have noticed that mothers who put lots of time and energy into a career, and then decide to stay home, may have trouble shutting off their natural competitive instincts. If they make you uncomfortable, find another friend to compare notes with.

HEAL FIRST

The demands of pregnancy, childbirth, and a new high maintenance family member can take a toll on your body, marriage, and lifestyle. The first weeks are the toughest. Your body is still healing and you may still look pregnant. Feeding is getting established, sleep patterns are erratic; everything is new. Factor in normal postpartum hormonal changes, and it's no wonder you're exhausted. Try to be patient and gentle with yourself. You can't be an effective parent unless you tend to your own needs, too. In time you can regain a slimmer body. The baby will eventually sleep through the night. Your newly configured family will become more functional. Try to heal first, then get organized and motivated to get back on top of your game.

Talking Together

Don't lose the interests and talents that make you who you are. You don't have to sacrifice everything, but you do have to prioritize. If you both agree, "We want to stay in shape," plan ahead together to make it happen, despite time pressures. Exercise pays dividends in body image and mental health (endorphins) and, surprisingly, will reduce fatigue. Keep exercise moderate, however. Excessive workouts may diminish your milk supply. Negotiate issues such as, "Can I still have a poker night out (or a Tuesday night tennis game or go to my pottery class)?"

If you feel isolated or cooped up, talk with your spouse about your life together. Both of you may feel the same way. You do need to avoid crowds to protect your infant from illness in the first two months, but that doesn't mean you have to be housebound. Fresh air is exhilarating. Families are incredibly mobile today. Babies go everywhere.

Realize, too, that a new mother may have the blues at this time. Talk together about mood swings and other behaviors that can cause friction between you and understand how blues differ from signs of postpartum depression.

CHAPTER 17

A Year to Remember

This chapter covers:

- What you've learned as a parent
- Looking ahead to baby's second year
- Contemplating another child
- Recognizing your strengths: a quiz

As you look back at the first year of your baby's life, you may be amazed at the ups and downs. Most parents go from enormous excitement and wonder at the miracle of birth to something resembling post-traumatic stress disorder. Once the euphoria of childbirth wears off, you now face sleepless nights, a language of crying you may not understand, daunting diaper changes, and worry, worry, worry. But after a few stress-filled weeks, you begin to get the hang of it. Amazingly, the baby is growing and gaining weight. You know what each cry means most of the time. You can change a diaper with one hand. You and your partner have learned to navigate chore assignments. Hopefully, you have a better sense of the work/home life issues that never get fully resolved, and your body is regaining its pre-pregnancy shape with lots of effort. Your baby continues to change and challenge you, but the journey is pretty amazing.

Here is a list of the "Top Ten Things Nobody Told You About" (or maybe they did but it didn't sink in):

1. Parenting is really, really hard.

2. Sometimes you wish you were not a parent.

3. Most of the time you cannot believe how much you love your baby.

4. Parenting requires lots of dollars.

5.   No matter what child care option you pick, you will never be totally satisfied.

6.   It is good that fathers are more involved today. Taking turns is a good thing!

7.   There are many ways to be a good parent.

8.   Sometimes you have to make it up as you go along.

9.   First you panic, but you do learn to cope.

10. Parenting humbles you—and enriches your life.

You can probably add discoveries of your own. Go ahead and do so. In fact, why not read this list together with your partner, share some laughs as well as insights, and feel good about what you've both learned and accomplished.

WHAT NEXT YEAR HOLDS

A whole new series of challenges await you in the next year of your baby's life, but you're going to be more savvy and confident about handling them. The second year is an exciting time for growth and development. Children start to talk and understand most language. They explore a wider environment, which adds a new threat of accidents and the need for accident prevention. Toddlers who were chubby when they started walking often shed a lot of baby weight as they grow into their bodies. But often they maintain a little belly.

This is a more active parenting stage than the passive parenting in the first twelve months, when babies sleep and eat much of the day. The constant vigilance required now will test your energy. Toddlers are always on the move. They're up and start weaning from two naps to one. The increase in awake time is a big adjustment that is fun, yet also exhausting.

A toddler may go on a food strike and eat so little that you obsess about starvation. Some children literally live on air. They are just too busy to eat and have become very finicky. Difficult as it may be, it's important to avoid pushing food into your child because that's how kids adopt a macaroni-and-cheese diet that's hard to break.

Children who have been very good sleepers may wake up again in the second year. All of us wake at night periodically, but babies want to know where you are. Usually it's separation anxiety. If you take them out of the crib at that time, you're going down a dark path (unless there's something amiss, such as a dirty diaper or a fever). Whining, which can be worse than crying, also emerges during the second year. Children start to want their independence, but they also want you. They're torn and get cranky.

Toward the end of the second year, especially as you head into toilet training, many children develop constipation. I advise parents to be vigilant about painful pooping, which can lead to withholding stool. Once established, this becomes a tough problem to solve; you can head it off with a stool softener. Your toddler may be ready for toilet training at two years or earlier although many children are closer to three in our culture.

BABY'S BEHAVIOR—AND YOURS

Discipline is not an issue until the middle and end of the second year when toddlers start to behave more provocatively. It's more than just exploring or being playful; they are testing limits. How will you and your partner handle it? Did your parents spank you? Is spanking acceptable for your offspring? If she is about to put a hand on a hot stove, do you slap it? Some people do; it's instinctual, as when a child runs out in the road. Parents are horrified and scared. How do you feel about yelling at the baby? Get a sense of how you want to cope with such situations and whether it's a case of "We're never going to do that." Talking it out can help check your own behavior in provocative situations.

What role do you want praise to play in your family? Do you praise every little thing your daughter says or does? Or will you be discriminating to prepare her for a more realistic view of life where she is not the center of the universe? Set the tone early to head off conflict later. You and your partner don't necessarily have to agree. If one of you comes from an abusive family, you may say, "I want my son to think he's the best," and that might be okay. Did you grow up in a large family where you got praise and attention only where you could find it? Can you allow your child to fail and learn from it?

What is your attitude toward manners, such as not interrupting people, which teaches children their place in the family? My father used to say, "Manners aren't for the child; they're for everyone else around the children." It's important for children to learn about respecting others (no hitting!), making a good impression, and being your best self. You want to arm your child with the skills to navigate the playground, at the table, and in the life that awaits him. Children who don't learn these things when they're little grow up and wonder why they don't have friends and aren't called back for second job interviews.

DO YOU WANT ANOTHER CHILD?

One of the issues most parents grapple with during the first year is "Should we have another child, and if so, when?" Unless finances are a major issue, couples do seem to replicate their own families of origin if they enjoyed the experience. I grew up in a family with four children, and I had four kids. As I was writing this book, my own daughter gave birth to her third child, a boy. The decision was easy in her case. She grew up in a household with three brothers and wanted more than two children. Whether she'll go for a fourth remains to be seen.

Four children might seem overwhelming if you grew up an only child or had one sibling. For me (and my daughter), four is normal and comfortable. But families with one child lavish a lot of attention on that child. Adults who are "onlys" might feel they couldn't give enough attention to more than one because that's what they got.

A lot of people choose to have only one child because both parents are working or they can't physically have another baby. Second child infertility is more common than people realize. Many parents are also older than those in past generations. They may have had infertility problems with a first baby and be unable to have a second or unwilling to go through the emotional rollercoaster once again. There are wonderful youngsters that come from big and small families, and opportunities abound today for only children to be socialized early in day care, preschool, and play groups. Learning to share and be stimulated by other children becomes a nonissue.

SPACING

If you do plan on another baby, how long should you wait before becoming pregnant again? This is a personal decision with no right answer. In the 1980s, a popular book by psychologist Burton White advocated for three-year spacing between babies. This recommendation is no longer in vogue as life has changed dramatically since then. In primitive societies, babies are naturally spaced about every two years as their mothers breastfeed almost constantly for a year (the only way that breastfeeding works as a contraceptive). Obviously, the more fully recovered you are from your previous pregnancy, the better your next pregnancy will feel.

Some parents opt for close spacing. One thirty-six-year-old working mother is glad she spaced her children (now five months and eighteen months) thirteen months apart because "It's over. Otherwise it would be a long drawn out parenting period." She and her husband feel their eighteen-month-old daughter also has no jealousy toward the baby at this age. "Although she may lift up her brother's eyelids when he's sleeping, she's curious and doesn't mean to hurt him."

Another working mom, age thirty, feels differently about a sibling right now for her eleven-month-old. "It isn't really possible to have another one now. I couldn't take the time off at work, and financially we aren't in a place to have a second one yet. We won't be for a few years," she says.

MIND YOUR MARRIAGE, NOURISH YOUR CORE

In the first year, parents' concerns focus on feeding, sleeping (or not), monitoring development, and avoiding infection. But other issues surface around these concerns. You and your partner have undoubtedly had skirmishes about problems you never had to confront before, such as: Is everybody doing his share? Are we in sync with letting the baby cry at times? Are other family members intruding with unwanted advice? Am I losing my identity? Will we ever have time for each other again? Is the child running the household and consuming our lives? Do I want a nanny living in our home?

There are no easy answers to such questions, but it is important to air your feelings—both good and bad—with one another. Maybe it's "Why do I always have to be the one to call the babysitter?" or "You always want to stay home. Why can't we go to Bill's wedding?" Sad to say, I have seen too many couples with young children get divorced. Don't wait until a rift is too large to repair. Sometimes parents are ashamed to air negative feelings about parenting because they know they are lucky and blessed to have a healthy baby. But if these feelings are hidden, they will emerge in other ways. You might be surprised to know how many other parents have experienced the very same feelings. Nobody ever said having a baby is unmitigated joy. And if they did, they were wrong. Parenting is a constant and exhausting balancing act.

FORGET PERFECTION

In a wonderful passage in John Grogan's book, *Marley and Me*, Grogan's wife, Jen, is despondent over a waterlogged and now dead dieffenbachia plant. "I can't even keep a stupid houseplant alive. I mean, how hard is that? . . . If I can't keep a houseplant alive, how am I ever going to keep a baby alive?" she asks.

Most new parents feel inadequate, too. They're daunted by their new responsibilities. As you've discovered, however, you can manage the job. Whether or not you're the perfect parent is another matter. In my experience, such a person doesn't exist. Everyone—and I do mean everyone—brings different strengths and challenges to parenting. Unless you accept your abilities, you're likely to continually feel you're failing or falling short. The task is to be a "good enough" parent, not "super mom."

WHO'S IN CHARGE?

Try not to have everything revolve around the baby. Children are important, but so are you. Babies do much better as part of the team rather than stars of a child-obsessed household. Don't let your child run the show or you can face long-term repercussions.

I've found that parents who can't bear to say no to a baby crying are the same ones who will have trouble

What Are Your Strengths?

Take an inventory of the strengths you do have, rather than dwell on what you think is missing. Check the ones that apply.

I'm good at:

- ❐ Calming the baby
- ❐ Being patient
- ❐ Cuddling with the baby
- ❐ Singing to the baby
- ❐ Playing with the baby
- ❐ Showing affection to the baby
- ❐ Throwing birthday parties for the baby
- ❐ Keeping the house relatively clean and organized
- ❐ Setting limits for the baby
- ❐ Getting the baby outdoors
- ❐ Teaching the baby new skills such as throwing a ball
- ❐ Communicating with the nanny, day care workers, or family members who babysit
- ❐ Taking control of a crisis (such as an injury to the baby or very high fever)
- ❐ Researching baby-related health information, resources, etc.

We're all good at some of these, but I don't know anyone who is good at all of them. How about you? Why not ask your partner and/or a friend with a baby to check the list and compare answers with yours. It's a great way to start an important discussion, get you both thinking, and build confidence at the same time. You may find that others think you're too modest about your self-assessment.

setting limits later, such as not allowing a four-year-old to crawl into their bed every night at 2:00 a.m., or insisting on time outs when children lose control, or grounding a teenager. I've always admired parents who can set limits firmly and effectively. You can explain your reason when the child has calmed. Remember you are the adults.

WELCOME TO YOUR NEW WORLD

You started the last year awed by the new life in your family. After twelve months your baby has grown and changed, and so have you.

I remember one father who worried that his one-month-old daughter was not making eye contact yet. Was she autistic? It is easy to dwell on milestones and possible disorders. This is what life is like with a first child. If you have a second or third baby, you can probably avoid some of these worries because you've been there. Hopefully you'll have more perspective if your neighbor's child walks or talks a lot earlier than your baby.

You now know that parenting is filled with change and uncertainty. Expect to make mistakes, analyze them, and move on. Try to make informed decisions, stay educated, but use information wisely. Most of all love your baby and enjoy this year of life!

Acknowledgments

I became a pediatrician because I enjoy children and interacting with families—and writing this book for parents has been a uniquely rewarding experience. It is also exciting when you discover a partner who complements you. In this case, I am not talking about my spouse, but rather my writing partner, Florence Isaacs. We've worked closely together as a team to produce a book that we hope will make this first year of your baby's life less confusing and stressful and more fun. We are both grateful to our editor Mary Norris, whose wise guidance has been invaluable, and to our agent, the intrepid Linda Konner. I also thank Julie Silver, MD, Chief Editor of Harvard Health Publications, without whose support this book would not have been possible.

Thanks to my family, of course, and to all the children—my own and the many patients who have taught me so much over the years.

—Victoria Rogers McEvoy, MD

Collaborating on a book can be a difficult balancing act. Fortunately, I worked with Vicky McEvoy, who is brilliant, kind, and fun—and made the process of creating this book a joy. I also thank six-month-old Joshua Harvey Isaacs, my first grandchild and the light of my life. He was born as we worked on this project and made the book come alive for me.

—Florence Isaacs

Resources

GENERALLY HELPFUL WEB SITES AND HOTLINES

American Academy of Family Physicians, www.aafp.org

American Academy of Pediatrics, www.aap.com

American Academy of Obstetricians and Gynecologists, www.acog.org

Centers for Disease Control, www.cdc.gov

Home Safety Council, www.homesafetycouncil.org

March of Dimes, www.marchofdimes.com; E-mail: askus@marchof
dimes.com

MedlinePlus, www.medlineplus.gov

National Center for Complementary and Alternative Medicine, www.nc
cam.nih.gov

National Institute of Child Health and Development, www.nichd.nih
.gov

National Institute of Mental Health, www.nimh.nih.gov

Pathways Awareness Foundation, www.pathwaysawareness.org;
1-800-326-8154

U.S. Department of Health and Human Services Office on Women's
Health, www.womenshealth.gov: Hotline: 1-800-994-9662

WebMD, www.children/webmd.com

BOOKS

Baby Signs, Linda Acredolo, PhD and Susan Goodwyn, PhD (McGraw-
Hill, 2007)

*Becoming a Family: Promoting Healthy Attachments with Your
Adopted Child,* Lark Eshleman, PhD (Taylor Trade Publishing,
2006)

Consumer Reports Best Baby Products 10th Edition, Sandra Gordon
and the Editors of *Consumer Reports* (Consumer Reports)

The Fussy Baby Book, William Sears, MD and Martha Sears, RN (Little
Brown and Company, 1996)

It's a Boy!, Michael Thompson, PhD (Ballantine Books, 2009)

Juggling Twins, Meghan Regan-Loomis (Sourcebooks, Inc., 2008)

Mothering Multiples, Karen Kerkhoff Gromada (La Leche League
    International, 2007)
The Premature Baby Book, James Sears, Martha Sears, Robert Sears,
    William Sears (Sears Parenting Library)
Raising Baby Green, Alan Greene, MD (Jossey-Bass, 2007)

SPECIFIC BABY CONCERNS

Allergies

"Timing is Everything When it Comes to Childhood Asthma." November
    21, 2008. www.newswise.com/articles/view/546740/?sc=dwhr;xy
    =5001381

Breastfeeding

American Academy of Breastfeeding Medicine, www.bfmed.org

"An Easy Guide to Breastfeeding," U.S. Department of Health and
    Human Services Office on Women's Health, www.womenshealth
    .gov

CDC twenty-four-hour breastfeeding hotline, 800-CDC-INFO (232-
    4636), cdcinfo@cdc.gov

"Frequently Asked Questions Breastfeeding," www.womens
    healthgov/FAQ/breastfeeding.cfm

La Leche League International, www.llli.org, Toll-free line: 1-800-525-
    3243

National Breastfeeding Hotline, www.womenshealth.gov, 1-800-994-
    9662

Child Care

"Choosing Quality Child Care: What's Best for Your Family," American
    Academy of Pediatrics, www.healthychildcare.org

National Association for Family Child Care, 1-800-359-3817, www
    .nafcc.org

Crying

"Colic," University of Virginia Health System, www.healthsystem.virginia
    .edu/uvahealth/adult_pediatrics/colic.cfm?printfriendly=1&

Day-to-Day Baby Care

"Travel Safety Tips," American Academy of Pediatrics, www.aap.org/
    advocacy/releases/travelsafetytips.cfm

Development

"Assure the Best for your Baby's Physical Development," Brochure
    from Pathways Awareness Foundation, www.pathwaysawareness
    .org; Parent-answered toll-free number: 1-800-955-CHILD (2445)

"Developmental Milestones," CDC Centers for Disease Control and Prevention, National Center on Birth Defects and Developmental Disabilities, www.cdc.gov/ncbddd/actearly/milestones

"Hearing Milestones in Infants/Toddlers," Child Link, The University of Maine, www.umaine.edu/link/HearMilestones.htm

Food and Nutrition

FDA toll-free hotline on storing and handling liquid or solid food for babies 888-SAFEFOOD (733-3663)

"Feeding Your 4–7-Month Old," *Kids Health,* Nemours Foundation, www.kidshealth.org/parent/nutrition_fit/nutrition/feed47m.html

"Feeding Your 8–12-Month Old," *Kids Health,* Nemours Foundation, www.kidshealth.org/parent/nutrition_fit/nutrition/feed812m.html

McEvoy, Vicky, MD "Can babies be obese?" July 1, 2008; www.gather .com/viewArticle/Dr. McEvoy

Health Information

"20 Things to Know about Evaluating Medical Resources on the Web," NCCAM Publication No. 142, NCCAM Clearinghouse, 1-888-644-6226, info@nccam.nih.gov

Illness

American Urological Association, Inc., aua@auanet.org, 1-866-746-4282 or 410-689-3700, www.urologyhealth.org

Eunice Kennedy Shriver National Institute of Child Health and Human Development Information Resource Center, www.nichd.nih.gov, 800-370-2943, E-mail: nichdinformationresourcecenter@mail .nih.gov

McEvoy, Vicky, MD, "Fever in Babies," March 2, 2009, www.gather .com/viewArticle.jsp?articleId=281474977611986&nav=Namespace

McEvoy, Vicky, MD, "Roseola: A Viral Illness that Causes Fever, Rash," June 2, 2008, www.gather.com/viewArticle.jsp?articleId=2814749 77359529&nav=Namespace

McEvoy, Vicky, MD, "The Stomach Flu in Babies: What to Do about Vomiting and Diarrhea," December 8, 2008, www.gather.com/ view Article.jsp?articleId=281474977529710&nav=Namespace

McEvoy, Vicky, MD, "When Your Baby Is Weeping Tears, But Not Crying," August 11, 2008, www.gather.com/viewArticle.jsp?article Id=281474977418865&nav=Namespace

Injuries and Accidents

American College of Emergency Physicians, www.acep.org/Patients
.aspx

"Choking Rescue Procedure (Heimlich Maneuver—Baby Younger
Than 1 Year)," www.children.webmd.com/guide/choking-rescue-
procedure-baby-younger-than-1-year

"CPSC Reminds Parents of Drowning Dangers Inside the Home," www
.cpsc.gov/cpscpub/prerel/prhtml08 /08417.html

Home Safety Council, www.homesafetycouncil.org/Safety Guide

Pee, Poop, Spit-Ups

McEvoy, Vicky, MD, "Constipation in Babies," September 15, 2008,
www.gather.com/viewArticle/McEvoy

McEvoy, Vicky, MD, "The Stomach Flu in Babies: What to Do about
Vomiting and Diarrhea," December 8, 2008, www.gather.com/
viewArticle/Dr.McEvoy

"What Can I Do If My Baby Gets Diaper Rash?" AAP Parenting Corner
Q&A: Diaper Rash, www.aap.org/publiced/br_diaperrash.htm

Personality

McEvoy, Vicky, MD, "Personality Types in Babies," November 10, 2008,
www.gather.com/viewArticle/Dr.McEvoy

Sleep

Back to Sleep Campaign, 1-800-CRIB (2742)

The Juvenile Products Manufacturers Association, www.jpma.org

National SIDS and Infant Death Resource Center, www.sidscenter.org

www.nichd.nih.gov/SIDS

Taking Care of Yourself

Hotline on depression during and after pregnancy, womenshealth.gov;
1-800-994-9662

Postpartum Education for Parents, (805) 564-3888; www.sbpep.org

Postpartum Support International, (805) 967-7636

Bibliography

CHAPTER 1: SLEEP

Bedtimes
Mindell, J. A., A. Sadeh, B. Wiegand, T. H. How, and D. Y. T. Goh, (in press). "Cross-Cultural Differences in Infant and Toddler Sleep." *Sleep Medicine,* (2008).

Safety
"The Catch with Co-Sleepers." http://blogs.consumerreports.org/baby/2007/04.

Coleman-Phox, Kimberly, Roxana Odouli, and De-Kun Li. "Use of a Fan During Sleep and the Risk of Sudden Infant Death Syndrome." *Archives of Pediatrics and Adolescent Medicine* 162, no. 10 (October 2008): 963–68.

Hauck, F. R., O. O. Omojokun, and M. S. Siadaty. "Do Pacifiers Reduce the Risk of Sudden Infant Death Syndrome? A meta-analysis." *Pediatrics* 116, no. 5 (November 2005): 716–23.

Roffwarg, Howard P., Joseph N. Muzio, and William C. Dement. "Ontogenic Development of Human Sleep-Dream Cycle." *Science* 152, no. 3722 (April 29, 1966): 604–19.

"Safe Sleep for Your Baby: Ten Ways to Reduce the Risk of Sudden Infant Death Syndrome (SIDS)." National Institute of Child Health and Human Development. www.nichd.nih.gov/publications/pubs/safe_sleep_gen.cfm.

Shapiro-Mendoza, Carrie K., Melissa Kimball, Kay M. Tomashek, Robert N. Anderson, and Sarah Blanding. "US Infant Mortality Trends Attributable to Accidental Suffocation and Strangulation in Bed from 1984 through 2004: Are Rates Increasing?" *Pediatrics* 123 no. 2 (February 2009): 533–39.

SIDS
American Academy of Pediatrics Policy Statement, "The Changing Concept of Sudden Infant Death Syndrome: Diagnostic Coding Shifts, Controversies Regarding the Sleeping Environment and New Variables to Consider in Reducing Risk" *Pediatrics* 116 no. 5 (November 2005). Statement of reaffirmation: *Pediatrics 123 no. 1/Jan.* 2009: http://aappolicy.aappublications.org/cgi/content/abstract/pediatrics;116/5/1245.

CHAPTER 2: BREASTFEEDING

General Findings

"Breastfeeding in the United States: Findings from the National Health and Nutrition Examination Survey, 1999-2006." NCHS Data Brief, Number 5, April 2008. Centers for Disease Control and Prevention. www.cdc.gov/nchs/data/databriefs/db05.htm.

"Research on Breastfeeding." National Institute of Child Health and Human Development, September 15, 2006. www.nichd.nih.gov/womenshealth/research/pregbirth/breastfeed.cfm.

Pumps

"Breast Pumps." *Consumer Reports*. www.consumerreports.org/cro/babies-kids/baby-toddler/eating-and-sleeping/breastpumps/breast-pumps-1105/overview.

Storing Breast Milk

"Breastfeeding Report Card." 2009: www.cdc.gov/BREASTFEEDING/DATA/report_card.htm.

"Proper Handling and Storage of Human Milk." Centers for Disease Control, May 22, 2007. www.cdc.gov/breastfeeding/recommendations/handling_breastmilk.htm.

Spencer, Jeanne P., Luis S. Gonzalez III, and Donna J. Barnhart. "Medications in the Breast-Feeding Mother." *American Family Physician,* July 1, 2001.

"Wet-Nursing in France," "Wet-Nursing in England," "Wet Nursing in Germany," "Wet-Nursing in the United States," *Encyclopedia of Children and Childhood in History and Society.* www.faqs.org/childhood/Th-W/Wet-Nursing.html.

CHAPTER 3: FOOD AND NUTRITION

Food Safety

"Once Baby Arrives: Food Safety for Moms-to-Be." U.S. Food and Drug Administration Center for Food Safety and Applied Nutrition. www.fda.gov/Food/ResourcesForYou/consumers/.../ucm089629.html.

High Chairs

"High chairs." *Consumer Reports*. www.consumerreports.org/cro/babies-kids/baby-toddler/eating-and-sleeping/high-ch.

Mayr, J. M., U. Seebacher, G. Schimpl, and F. Fiala. "Highchair Accidents." *Acta Paediatr* 88, no. 3 (March 1999): 319–22. www.ncbi.nlm.nih.gov/pubmed/10229045.

Organic Foods

Magkos, F., F. Arvaniti, and A. Zampelas. "Organic Food or Food for Thought? A Review of the Evidence." *International Journal of Food Sciences and Nutrition* 54, no. 5 (September 2003): 357–71.

"Organic Production/Organic Food: Information Access Tools," USDA, June 2007. www.usda.gov/afsic/pubs/ofp/ofp.shtml.

Tasiopoulou, S., A. M. Chiodini, F. Vellere, and S. Visentin. "Results of the Monitoring Program of Pesticide Residues in Organic Food of Plant Origin in Lombardy (Italy)." *Journal of Environmental Science and Health Part B* 42, no. 7 (Sept–Oct 2007): 835–41. www.ncbi.nlm.nih.gov/pubmed/17763041.

Solids

"Starting Solids: Nutrition Guide for Infants and Children 6 to 18 Months of Age." International Food Information Council, January 2005. www.ific.org/publications/brochures/solidsbroch.cfm.

Water

"The Facts about Bottled Water." *Journal of the American Dental Association* 134 (September 2003): 1287.

"Fact Sheet on Questions about Bottled Water and Fluoride." October 31, 2008. www.cdc.gov/fluoridation/fact.../bottled_water.html.

Scelfo, Julie. "F.D.A. to Reconsider Plastic Bottle Risk," *New York Times,* December 23, 2008. www.nytimes.com/2008/12/24/dining/24chem.html?ref=dining.

Weight

Taveras, Elsie, and Matthew Gillman. "Infant Weight Gain Linked to Childhood Obesity." *Pediatrics* 123, no. 4 (April 2009). www.newswise.com/articles/view/550477/?sc=dwhr;xy=5001381.

CHAPTER 4: CRYING

Colic

"Colic and crying." *MedlinePlus,* December 1, 2008. www.nlm.nih.gov/MEDLINEPLUS/ency/article/000978.htm.

Hill, D. "Effects of a Low Allergen Maternal Diet on Colic Among Breastfed Infants: A Randomized, Controlled Trial." *Pediatrics,* November 7, 2005; vol. 116: e709–e715.

Jobe, Alan H. "The Effects of Probiotics on Feeding Tolerance, Bowel Habits, and Gastrointestinal Motility in Preterm Newborns." *Journal of Pediatrics* 152, no. 6 (June 2008): A1.

Savino, F., et al. "Lactobacillus reuteri (American Type Culture Collection Strain 55730) Versus Simethicone in the Treatment of Infantile Colic: A Prospective Randomized Study." *Pediatrics* 119, no. 1 (January 2007), e124–e130.

Savino, F. et al. "Reduction of crying episodes owing to infantile colic: A randomized controlled study of a new infant formula"; *Eur J Clin Nutr,* 60:1304,2006.

Folk Remedies

"FDA Issues Advisory on Star-Anise 'Teas.'" *FDA News,* September 10, 2003.

"Folk Remedies Common Cause of Lead Poisoning," Associated Press, January 22, 2008. www.msnbc.msn.com/id/22782271.

"Lead Poisoning from Folk Home Remedies." Virginia Department of Health, Division of Environmental Epidemiology, January 24, 2008. www.vdh.virginia.gov/Epidemiology/DEE.

Smitherman, Lynn C., James Janisse, and Ambika Mathur. "The Use of Folk Remedies Among Children in an Urban Black Community: Remedies for Fever, Colic, and Teething." *Pediatrics* 115, no. 3 (March 2005): e297-c304. www.pediatrics.org/cgi/content/full/115 /3/e297.

Picking Up

"For Crying Out Loud—Pick Up Your Baby," *Science Daily,* Queensland University of Technology, October 28, 2006. www.sciencedaily.com/releases/2006/10/061027184248.htm.

Probiotics

Johannes, Laura. "Bug Crazy: Assessing the Benefits of Probiotics." *Wall Street Journal,* January 13, 2009, p. D6.

Signing

Acredolo, Linda, and Susan Goodwin. "Symbolic gesturing in normal infants." *Child Development* 1988, 59, 450–466. www.babysigns.com.

"Navy Child Development Programs Teach 'Baby Signs.'" Fleet and Family Readiness Marketing, Commander, Navy Installations Command, March 15, 2007. www.news.navy.mil/search/display.asp?story_id=28316.

Thompson, Rachel H., Nicole M. Cotnoir-Bichelman, Paige M. McKerchar, Trista L. Tate, and Kelly A. Dancho. "Enhancing Early Communication Through Infant Sign Training," *Journal of Applied Behavior Analysis* 40, no. 1 (Spring 2007): 15–23.

CHAPTER 5: PEE, POOP, AND SPIT-UPS

Diapers
Paul, Pamela. "Diapers Go Green," *Time,* January 10, 2008. www.time
.com/time/printout/0,8816,1702357.00.html.

Toilet Training
Rugolotto, Simone, and Min Sun. "Toilet Training." *Pediatrics* 113, no. 1
(January 2004): pp. 180–81 www.pediatrics.aappublications.org/
cgi/content/full/113/1/180.

Urine
Thornton, Stephen L., MD. "Pediatrics, Urinary Tract Infections and
Pyelonephritis." emedicine.medscape.com/article/804866-
overview.

CHAPTER 6: GROWTH AND DEVELOPMENT

Autism
Valeo, Tom. "No Vaccine Link Found." *BrainWork* (March–April 2008): 7.

Language Development
"Carnegie Mellon Study: Adults' Baby Talk Helps Infants Learn To
Speak." *ScienceDaily* (March 31, 2005). www.sciencedaily.com/
releases/2005/03/050329143741.htm.

Milestones
Berger, Kathleen Stassen. *The Developing Person through Childhood
and Adolescence.* New York: Worth Publishers, 2006.

Tests
Beck, Melinda. "How's Your Baby? Recalling the Apgar Score's
Namesake." *Wall Street Journal, Personal Journal,* May 26, 2009:
D1.

CHAPTER 7: BABIES' BODIES

Birth Weight
Madan A., S. Holland, J. E. Humbert, and W. E. Benitz. "Racial
Differences in Birth Weight of Term Infants in a Northern
California Population." *Journal of Perinatology* 22, no. 5
(July–August 2002): 339–40. www.ncbi.nlm.nih.gov/pubmed/
11948387?dopt.

Circumcision

"Should Your Son Be Circumcised?" Associated Press, June 15, 2006, Fact File.

Strabismus

"Strabismus (Cross-Eyes)" FamilyDoctor.org. www.familydoctor.org/online/famdocen/home/children/parents/special/birth/309.html.

CHAPTER 8: DAY-TO-DAY BABY CARE

Safety

"Child Passenger Safety." National Highway Traffic and Safety Administration. www.nhtsa.dot.gov.

TV and DVDs

Christakis, Dimitri A., Jill Gilkerson, Jeffrey A. Richards, Frederick J. Zimmerman, Michelle M. Garrison, Dongxin Xu, Sharmistha Gray, and Umit Yapanel. "Audible Television and Decreased Adult Words, Infant Vocalizations, and Conversational Turns." *Archives of Pediatrics & Adolescent Medicine* 163, no. 6 (June 2009).

Mendelson, Alan L., Samantha B. Berkule, Suzy Tomopoulos, Catherine S. Tamis-LeMonda, Harris S. Huberman, Jose Alvir, Penard P. Dreyer. "Infant Television and Video Exposure Associated with Limited Parent-Child Verbal Interactions in Low Socioeconomic Status Households." *Archives of Pediatrics & Adolescent Medicine* 162, no. 5 (May 2008). www.archpedi.ama-assn.org/cgi/content/abstract/162/5/411.

Nyhan, Paul. "40% of babies watch TV, UW study finds." Seattle, P-I. www.seattlepi.com/local/314676_babytube08.html.

Schwarz, Joel. "Baby DVDs, Videos May Hinder, Not Help Infants' Language Development," *University of Washington News,* August 7, 2007. www.uwnews.org/article.asp?articleid=35898.

Zimmerman, Frederick J., Dimitri A. Christakis, and Andrew N. Meltzoff. "Associations between Media Viewing and Language Development in Children Under Age 2 Years." *The Journal of Pediatrics* 151, no. 4 (October 2007): 364–68. www.jpeds.com/article/PIIS0022347607 004477.

CHAPTER 9: IMMUNIZATIONS

Flu Vaccine

"AAP Policy Statement Calls for All Children, Age 6 Months through 18 Years, to Receive Influenza Vaccine," November 3, 2008. www.cispimmunize.org/ill/Flu/Influenza.

Goldstein, Jacob. "In the War Against Flu's Mutants, a Big Ally Is Weakened." *Wall Street Journal,* March 3, 2009.

MMR Vaccine

McNeil Jr., Donald G. "Book Is Rallying Resistance to the Antivaccine Crusade" *New York Times,* January 13, 2009, p. D1.

"Why Do People Think that Vaccines Can Cause Autism?" National Institute of Child Health and Human Development , August 15, 2006. www.nichd.nih.gov/publications/pubs/upload/autism/MMR .pdf.

"Why Do So Many Doctors and Scientists Believe that the MMR Vaccine Does Not Cause Autism?" National Institute of Child Health and Human Development, February 1, 2009. www.nichd .nih.gov/publications/pubs/autism/mmr/sub3.cfm.

SIDS and Vaccines

"Sudden Infant Death Syndrome (SIDS) and Vaccines." Centers for Disease Control and Prevention. www.cdc.gov/vaccinesafety/ updates/sids_faq.htm.

Vaccination Schedule

"Recommended Immunity Schedule for Persons Aged 0 through 6 Years—United States 2009." www.CDC.gov/vaccines/recs/ schedules/downloads/child/.../09_0-6yrs.

Vaccinations and Autism

Doren, Jennifer Corbett. "Autism Study to Follow Pregnant Women," *Wall Street Journal,* June 9, 2009, p. D2.

Harris, Gardiner. "Court Hears More Claims of Vaccine-Autism Link," *New York Times,* May 13, 2008, p. A14.

McNeil, Donald G. "Court Finds No Link of Vaccine and Autism," *New York Times,* February 13, 2009, p. A16.

www.cdc.gov/ncbddd/autism/index.html

CHAPTER 10: ILLNESS

Febrile Seizures

"Febrile seizures." *MedlinePlus,* August 2, 2008. www.nlm.nih.gov/ medlineplus/ency/article/000980.htm.

Fliesler, Nancy. "Spinal Tap Unnecessary for Most Babies with Uncomplicated Febrile Seizures." *Harvard Science,* January 9, 2009. www.harvardscience.harvard.edu/medicine-health/topics/ pediatrics.

"What are febrile seizures?" *Consumer Reports Health,* June 9, 2008. www.consumerreports.org/health/conditions-and-treatments/ febrile-seizures.

Folk Remedies

Smitherman, Lynn C., James Janisse, and Ambika Mathur. "The Use of Folk Remedies Among Children in an Urban Black Community: Remedies for Fever, Colic, and Teething." *Pediatrics* 115 (2005): e297–c304.

RSV

"Respiratory Syncytial Virus (RSV)." March of Dimes' Pregnancy & Newborn Health Education Center, July 2006. www.marchof dimes.com/printableArticles/298_9546.asp.

UTIs

"Urine Blockage in Newborns." February 2006. www.kidney.niddk.nih .gov/kudiseases/pubs/newborns.

CHAPTER 11: INJURIES AND ACCIDENTS

Burns

Oesterreich, Lesia. "Is Your Baby Safe at Home? Part 2-Burns." Iowa State University, November 2003. www.nncc.org/Health/baby burns.html.

Drowning

Brenner, Ruth A., Ann C. Trumble, Gordon S. Smith, Eileen P. Kessler, and Mary D. Overpeck. "Where Children Drown, United States, 1995." *Pediatrics* 108, no. 1 (July 2001): 85–89.

"CPSC Reminds Parents of Drowning Dangers Inside the Home." September 30, 2008. www.cpsc.gov/cpscpub/prerel/prhtml08/ 08417.html.

Falls

"Is Your Baby Safe at Home? Part 3-Falls." Iowa State University Extension. www.nncc.org/Health/babyfalls.html.

Policy Statement: "Injuries Associated with Infant Walkers" *Pediatrics* 108, no. 3 (September 2001): 790–92. Reaffirmation of policy published on August 1, 2008.

"U.S. Government Should Ban Baby Walkers." Release April 8, 2004, American Academy of Pediatrics. www.aap.org/advocacy/ washing/New-Release_Press-Statements/04-08-04-Ban-Baby- Walkers.htm.

General Safety

Colino, Stacey. "How to accident-proof your kids." CNN.com. www.cnn
.site.printthis.clickability.com/pt/cpt?action=cpt&title=How+to+
accident-proof+.

"Is Your Baby Safe at Home? Part 4-Hazards." Iowa State University
Extension. www.nncc.org/Health/babyhazards.html.

www.homesafetycouncil.org/StartSafe/ss_baby_w001.asp.

Poisoning

Arnquist, Sarah. "Poison Control Centers May Be Budget Victims."
New York Times, June 30, 2009, p. D7.

Oesterreich, Lesia. "Is Your Baby Safe at Home? Part 1-Poison." www
.nncc.org/Health/babypoison.html.

Suffocation and Strangling

"Safety Tips for Sleeping Babies." U.S. Consumer Products Safety
Commission. www.cpsc.gov/cpscpub/pubs/203.html.

Shapiro-Mendoza, Carrie K., Melissa Kimball, Kay M. Tomashek, Robert
N. Anderson, and Sarah Blanding. "US Infant Mortality Trends
Attributable to Accidental Suffocation and Strangulation in Bed
from 1984 Through 2004: Are Rates Increasing?" *Pediatrics* 123,
no. 2 (February 2009): 533-39.

CHAPTER 12: ALLERGIES

"Daycare Protects Against Pediatric Asthma," release from American
Academy of Allergy, Asthma & Immunology (AAAAI), September
8, 2008.

Ely, Elissa. "House Dust Yields Clue to Asthma Roaches." *New York
Times,* April 2, 2009, p. D1.

"Food for Thought—Understanding Food Allergies in Kids."
Washington University in St. Louis, April 17, 2009. www.newswise
.com/articles/view/550925/?sc=sphr.

CHAPTER 13: HEALTH INFORMATION

Markoff, John. "Medical Web Searches and Escalating Fears," *New
York Times,* Nov. 25, 2008, p. B3.

Pew Internet & American Life Project: Online Life Report, 2003.

CHAPTER 14: WORK/CAREER

Child Care

"Child Care Factors Associated with Weight Gain in Infancy," July 7, 2008, *Archives of Pediatrics & Adolescent Medicine 162, no. 7 (2008)*: 627–33.

"Grandparents a Safe Source of Childcare." Johns Hopkins Bloomberg School of Public Health. www.newswise.com/articles/view/545914/?sc=mwtr;xy=5001381.

Shellenbarger, Sue. "Families Cut Back on Day Care as Costs—and Worries—Rise." *Wall Street Journal,* December 10, 2008, p. D1.

Maternity Leave

The Associated Press. "U.S. Stands Apart from Other Nations on Maternity Leave," *USA Today,* July 25, 2005. www.usatoday.com/news/health/2005-07-26-maternity-leave_x.htm.

Han, Wen-Jui, Christopher J. Ruhm, Jane Waldfogel, and Elizabeth Washbrook. "The Timing of Mothers' Employment after Childbirth." *Monthly Labor Review,* June 2008.

Shellenbarger, Sue. "Downsizing Maternity Leave: Employers Cut Pay, Time Off." *Wall Street Journal,* June 11, 2008.

Work Choices

Shellenbarger, Sue. "Does Avoiding a 9-to-5 Grind Make You a Target for Layoffs?" *Wall Street Journal,* April 22, 2009.

CHAPTER 15: MARRIAGE

Coontz, Stephanie. "Till Children Do Us Part." *New York Times,* February 5, 2009, p. A31.

University of Denver. "Children Take a Toll on Marital Bliss." *ScienceDaily,* April 8, 2009. www.sciencedaily.com/releases/2009/04/090408145351.htm.

CHAPTER 16: CARING FOR YOURSELF

McGovern, Pat, Bryan Dowd, Dwenda Gjerdingen, Cynthia Gross, Sally Kenney, Laurie Ukestad, David McCaffrey, and Ulf Lundberg.

"Postpartum Health of Employed Mothers 5 Weeks After Childbirth." *Annals of Family Medicine* 4, no. 2 (March 2006): 159–67.

"Understanding Postpartum Depression." *NIH News in Health,* December 2005. www.newsinhealth.nih.gov/December2005/docs/01features_02.htm.

Index